ARTIFICIAL INSEMINATION

Papers by
Richard B. Bourne, Jan Raboch, George W.
Matheson, William J. Curran, G. E. Seidel,
J. F. T. Griffin, J. W. MacPherson, J. P.
Frappell, John C. Ellery, John P. Hughes,
I. D. Killeen, R. J. Lightfoot, S. Salamon,
T. D. Quinlivan, Martin Sevoian, Patricia
Sarvella, J. B. K. Clark, Karl E. Nester,
M. Perek et al.

MSS Information Corporation
655 Madison Avenue, New York, N.Y. 10021

Library of Congress Cataloging in Publication Data
Main entry under title:

Artificial insemination.

    1. Artificial insemination--Addresses, essays,
lectures. 2. Artificial insemination, Human--
Addresses, essays, lectures. I. Bourne, Richard B.
[DNLM: 1. Insemination, Artificial--Collected
works. WQ 208 A791 1973]
SF105.5.A7   636.08'245   72-13433
ISBN 0-8422-7077-9

TABLE OF CONTENTS

CREDITS AND ACKNOWLEDGEMENTS

Bourne, Richard B.; William A. Kretzschmar; and John H. Esser, "Successful Artificial Insemination in a Diabetic with Retrograde Ejaculations," *Fertility and Sterility*, 1971, 22:275-277.

Clark, J.B.K., "Observations on the Dilution and Storage of Turkey Semen," *Veterinary Record*, 1969, 84:6-11.

Curran, William J., "Artificial Insemination," *Public Health and the Law*, 58:1460-1461.

Ellery, John C., "A Modified Equine Artificial Vagina for the Collection of Gel-Free Semen," *Journal of the American Veterinary Medical Association*, 1971, 158:765-766.

Frappell, J.P., "The Use of A.I. Centre Records in Applied Science," *Veterinary Record*, 1969, 84:381-385.

Griffin, J.F.T.; W.R. Nunn; and P.J. Hartigan, "An Immune Response to Egg-Yolk Semen Diluent in Dairy Cows," *Journal of Reproduction and Fertility*, 1971, 25:193-199.

Hughes, John P.; and Robert G. Loy, "Artificial Insemination in the Equine: A Comparison of Natural Breeding and Artificial Insemination of Mares Using Semen From Six Stallions," *Cornell Veterinarian*, 1970, 60:463-475.

Killeen, I.D.; and N.W. Moore, "Fertilization and Survival of Fertilized Eggs in the Ewe Following Surgical Insemination at Various Times after the Onset of Oestrus," *Australian Journal of Biological Sciences*, 1970, 23:1279-1287.

Killeen, I.D.; and N.W. Moore, "The Morphological Appearance and Development of Sheep Ova Fertilized by Surgical Insemination," *Journal of Reproduction and Fertility*, 1971, 24:63-70.

Killeen, I.D.; and N.W. Moore, "Transport of Spermatozoa, and Fertilization in the Ewe Following Cervical and Uterine Insemination Early and Late in Oestrus," *Australian Journal of Biological Sciences*, 1970, 23:1271-1277.

Lightfoot, R.J., "Studies on the Number of Ewes Joined per Ram for Flock Matings under Paddock Conditions: The Effect of Mating on Semen Characteristics," *Australian Journal of Agricultural Research*, 1968, 19:1043-1057.

Lightfoot, R.J.; and B.J. Restall, "Effects of Site of Insemination, Sperm Motility and Genital Tract Contractions on Transport of Spermatozoa in the Ewe," *Journal of Reproduction and Fertility*, 1971, 26:1-13.

Lightfoot, R.J.; and S. Salamon, "Fertility of Ram Spermatozoa Frozen by the Pellet Method: Transport and Viability of Spermatozoa within the Genital Tract of the Ewe," *Journal of Reproduction and Fertility*, 1970, 22:385-398.

Lightfoot, R.J.; and S. Salamon, "Fertility of Ram Spermatozoa Frozen by the Pellet Method: The Effects of Method of Insemination on Fertilization and Embryonic Mortality," *Journal of Reproductive Fertility*, 1970, 22:399-408.

Lightfoot, R.J.; and J.A.C. Smith, "Studies on the Number of Ewes Joined per Ram for Flock Matings under Paddock Conditions: Mating Behaviour and Fertility," *Australian Journal of Agricultural Research*, 1968, 19:1029-1042.

Macpherson, J.W., "Semen Placement Effects on Fertility in Bovines," *Journal of Dairy Science*, 1968, 51:807-808.

Matheson, George W.; Lars Carlborg; and Carl Gemzell, "Frozen Human Semen for Artificial Insemination," *American Journal of Obstetrics and Gynecology*, 1969, 104:495-501.

Nestor, Karl E.; and Keith I. Brown, "Method and Frequency of Artificial Insemination and Turkey Fertility," *Poultry Science*, 1968, 47:717-721.

Perek, M.; M. Elian; and E.D. Heller, "Bacterial Flora of Semen and Contamination of the Reproductive Organs of the Hen Following Artificial Insemination," *Research in Veterinary Science*, 1969, 10:127-132.

Quinlivan, T.D.; and T.J. Robinson, "Numbers of Spermatozoa in the Genital Tract after Artificial Insemination of Progestagen-Treated Ewes," *Journal of Reproduction and Fertility*, 1969, 19:73-86.

Raboch, Jan; and Z.D. Tomasek, "Therapeutic Donor Insemination — Results," *Journal of Reproduction and Fertility*, 1967, 14:421-425.

Salamon, S.; and R.J. Lightfoot, "Fertility of Ram Spermatozoa Frozen by the Pellet Method: The Effects of Insemination Technique, Oxytocin and Relaxin on Lambing," *Journal of Reproduction and Fertility*, 1970, 22:409-423.

Sarvella, Patricia, "Frequency of Parthenogenesis in Chickens after Insemination with Irradiated Sperm," *Radiation Research*, 1971, 46:186-191.

Seidel, G.E.; and R.H. Foote, "Motion Picture Analysis of Ejaculation in the Bull," *Journal of Reproduction and Fertility*, 1969, 20:313-317.

Sevoian, Martin, "Transmission of Type II (Marek's) Leukosis with Semen from Infected Roosters," *Poultry Science*, 1971, 50:1530-1532.

PREFACE

New technological advances in artificial insemination have been made in recent years and are already used by cattle breeders and in laboratory research. As the present collection shows, artificial insemination can be practiced in turkeys, rabbits, laboratory rodents and cats, as well as in the more traditional horses, pigs, sheep, and cows.

While also a useful and practical technique for humans, artificial insemination is, however, surrounded with psychological, social, legal, and medical problems. These topics are covered in this volume, representing the most important research published since 1967.

Artificial Insemination in Humans: Medical and Technical Aspects

SUCCESSFUL ARTIFICIAL INSEMINATION IN A DIABETIC WITH RETROGRADE EJACULATION

RICHARD B. BOURNE, M.D., WILLIAM A. KRETZSCHMAR, M.D., AND JOHN H. ESSER, M.D.

Retrograde ejaculation is an uncommon cause of infertility because it is usually iatrogenic and occurs in an older age group. The fact that it is also a complication of diabetes has been known since 1963.[1]

Ejaculation in man is usually mediated through higher centers, but it may be completely reflex. It has been noted that judicial hanging is often accompanied by ejaculation.[2] There are two stages in the ejaculatory process.[3] In the first or emission stage, rhythmic contractions expel the contents of the epididymis, vas deferens, seminal vesicle, and prostate into the prostatic urethra. This is probably mediated through the parasympathetic nervous system.[2, 4] The presence of semen in the prostatic urethra is believed to initiate the second stage, which involves relaxation of the external urethral sphincter, allowing the semen to flow into the bulbous urethra, and at the same time closure of the bladder neck to prevent regurgitation of semen into the bladder. Reflex contractions of the bulbocavernosus and ischiocavernosus muscles then propel the seminal fluid out through the urethra. In retrograde ejaculation the seminal fluid flows backward into the bladder, presumably due to failure of closure of the bladder neck.

METHOD

The patient is a 33-year-old man who has been diabetic since the age of 8 years and blind for the past 3 years. He was married 4 years ago and presented as an infertility problem. To his knowledge there has been no ejaculation since the age of 25 years, although orgasm has been normal.

The diagnosis of retrograde ejaculation was made by confirming the absence of an ejaculate in a condom after intercourse and then seeing spermatozoa in the postcoital urine specimen.

The menstrual periods of the patient's wife were very regular, and it was decided to inseminate her on the 11th and 13th days of her cycle. The technic used was basically the same as that described by Hotchkiss.[5] The bladder was first irrigated with 250 ml. of 5% dextrose in lactated Ringer's solution, and 2 ml. of the solution were left in the bladder prior to removal of the catheter. The patient was then allowed to ejaculate, and the specimen was obtained by having him void as soon as possible. If he had not been able to void, of course, the specimen would have to be obtained by catheterization. The voided specimen, usually about 10–30 ml., was then centrifuged at 3400 r.p.m. (Adams Sero-Fuge, Clay Adams, Division of Becton, Dickinson & Co. B-D, Parsippany, N.J.) for 3 min. and the sediment was inseminated in his wife.

This procedure was carried out eight times over a 6-month period without success. On several occasions the specimen revealed 25–50 sperm/high power field, but motility was uniformly poor. Examination of the uncentrifuged specimen also showed poor motility, and it was noted that the pH was always acid. Since it is well-known that the urine acidity is spermatocidal, the patient was alkalinized by giving him 6 0.6-gm. tablets of sodium bicarbonate the evening before and the morning of the insemination. The pH of the specimen then ranged from 7.0–7.5, and there was a marked improvement in sperm motility. The sediment now showed 50–100 actively motile sperm/high power field, and in January 1970 the patient's wife happily announced she was late for her period. On September 26, 1970 she gave birth to a normal healthy 7 lb. 12 oz. baby girl.

DISCUSSION

Retrograde ejaculation occurs when there is failure of the bladder neck to close during orgasm. There are two major iatrogenic causes of this. The first is incompetence of the bladder neck following surgical resection or repair for obstructive disease. Rieser[6] found that retrograde ejaculation occurred in 42% of cases following transurethral prostatectomy, and Ochsner[7] reported an incidence of 33% after bladder neck revision, either open or transurethral.

The second iatrogenic cause involves the fact that sympathetic nerves are responsible for closing the bladder neck during ejaculation. This was demonstrated in man by the classic studies of Learmonth[8] in 1931, and more recently by Kleeman,[9] who inserted a cystoscope into the dome of a dog's bladder and was able to observe the bladder neck close tightly during an intravenous infusion of epinephrine. He then observed a similar although slightly less marked effect from stimulation of the presacral nerve, and this occurred even during full parasympathetic stimulation using urecholine. He concluded that the bladder neck is under sympathetic control and that it is capable of closing even while the detrusor contracts.

It follows therefore that surgical removal of these sympathetic nerves or ganglia might result in failure of the bladder neck to close during ejaculation, and indeed, retrograde ejaculation has been reported to occur in 10%[10] to 64%[4] of cases following bilateral lumbar sympathectomy. Goligher[11] found a 39% incidence of retrograde ejaculation after abdominoperineal resections, and it has also been reported

after extensive retroperitoneal lymphadenectomy,[12] presumably due to damage of sympathetic nerves. Chemical sympathectomy can result in retrograde ejaculation, and Schirger and Gifford[13] found that this occurred in 23% of 22 men on guanethidine.

Noniatrogenic retrograde ejaculation may be congenital,[14] or due to trauma[15] or diabetes.[1, 16] The etiologic factor in diabetes is most likely the involvement of the sympathetic nerves to the bladder neck, since it has been shown that the sympathetic nervous system may be affected by diabetic neuropathy.[17, 18] Since Greene[19] has shown that sympathomimetic drugs have been of no avail in the treatment of this complication of diabetes, insemination of the semen after it has been recovered from the bladder remains the only mode of therapy. Artificial insemination in retrograde ejaculation has been successfully accomplished and reported seven times previously.[5, 6, 20, 21]

SUMMARY

This is the 8th reported case of successful artificial insemination in a patient with retrograde ejaculation, and the first in a diabetic.

Centrifugation of the seminal specimen did not adversely affect the spermatozoa, and at least in this case alkalinization of the patient was a valuable adjunct in improving the quality of the specimen.

REFERENCES

1. Greene, L. F., Kelalis, P. P., and Weeks, R. E. Retrograde ejaculation of semen due to diabetic neuropathy. *Fertil Steril 14:*617, 1963.
2. Potts, I. F. The mechanism of ejaculation. *Med J Aust 1:*495, 1957.
3. Masters, W. H., and Johnson, V. E. *Human Sexual Response.* Little, Brown, Boston, 1966, p. 212.
4. Retief, P. J. M. Physiology of micturition and ejaculation. *S Afr Med J 24:*509, 1950.
5. Hotchkiss, R. S., Pinto, A. B., and Kleegman, S. Artificial insemination with semen recovered from the bladder. *Fertil Steril 6:*37, 1955.
6. Rieser, C. The etiology of retrograde ejaculation

and a method for insemination. *Fertil Steril 12:* 488, 1961.

7. OCHSNER, M. G., BURNS, E., AND HENRY, H. H. Incidence of retrograde ejaculation following bladder neck revision as a child. *J Urol 104:*596, 1970.

8. LEARMONTH, J. R. A contribution to the neurophysiology of the urinary bladder in man. *Brain 54:*147, 1931.

9. KLEEMAN, F. J. The physiology of the internal urinary sphincter. *J Urol 104:*549, 1970.

10. ROSE, S. S. Investigation into sterility after lumbar ganglionectomy. *Brit Med J 1:*247, 1953.

11. GOLIGHER, J. C. Sexual function after excision of the rectum. *Proc Roy Soc Med 44:*824, 1951.

12. LEITER, E., AND BRENDLER, H. Loss of ejaculation following bilateral retroperitoneal lymphadenectomy. *J Urol 98:*375, 1967.

13. SCHIRGER, A., AND GIFFORD, R. W. Guanethidine, a new antihypertensive agent: Experience in the treatment of 36 patients with severe hypertension. *Proc Mayo Clin 37:*100, 1962.

14. GENNSER, G., OWMAN, T., AND WEHLIN, L. Significance of adrenergic innervation of the bladder outlet during ejaculation. *Lancet 1:*154, 1969.

15. SCHIRREN, C., KLOSTERHALFEN, H., AND KAUFMANN, J. Andrologic diagnosis: Retrograde ejaculation caused by an accident. *Z Haut Geschlechtskr 38:*344, 1965.

16. ELLENBERG, M., AND WEBER, H. Retrograde ejaculation in diabetic neuropathy. *Ann Intern Med 65:*1237, 1966.

17. ODEL, H. M., ROTH, G. M., AND KEATING, F. R. Autonomic neuropathy simulating the effects of sympathectomy as a complication of diabetes mellitus. *Diabetes 4:*92, 1955.

18. FAGERBERG, S-E., KOCK, N. G., PETERSÉN, I., AND STENER, I. Urinary bladder disturbances in diabetics. *Scand J Urol Nephrol 1:*19, 1967.

19. GREENE, L. F., AND KELALIS, P. P. Retrograde ejaculation of semen due to diabetic neuropathy. *J Urol 98:*693, 1968.

20. FISCHER, I. C., AND COATS, E. C. Sterility due to retrograde ejaculation of semen. *Obstet Gynec 4:* 352, 1954.

21. WALTERS, D., AND KAUFMAN, M. S. Sterility due to retrograde ejaculation of semen. *Amer J Obstet Gynec 78:*274, 1959.

THERAPEUTIC DONOR INSEMINATION—RESULTS

JAN RABOCH AND ZD. TOMÁŠEK

INTRODUCTION

Therapeutic donor insemination, AID, is in general a technically not too complicated gynaecological procedure which is performed in a supposedly fertile woman from andrologic indications, using semen of good quality. A rich literature of the complex problems involved in this procedure has been reviewed and appraised by Schellen (1957) and Beuerlein (1963). The results achieved by various authors in fairly large groups of patients treated by this method have been summarized in the report of Behrman (1959).

The authors of the present article agree with Kleegman (1954) who says that "Whether the procedure is good or bad should be decided on the results thereof" and "too many conclusions are based on phantasy or personal emotional attitudes". They now report on their experiences with AID and the results obtained in the course of 15 years with 219 sterile married couples.

MATERIALS

Therapeutic donor inseminations were performed in 219 women. The results of repeated seminal investigations of their husbands are summarized in Table 1.

Almost two-thirds of the men were repeatedly azoospermic. In those with obstruction we insisted that in the first place surgical correction of this state be attempted by vaso-epididymo-anastomosis. In nineteen men the number of spermatozoa was, in the majority of cases, less than 20 million/ml. Therapeutic donor insemination was performed in these cases only after therapy had failed to improve the seminology and when the married couple had remained sterile for at least 2 years. We proceeded in the same way in cases of severe oligozoospermia (less than 5 million spermatozoa/ml).

METHODS

As a rule, several months are needed for repeated seminological investigation of the husband, and at least three menstrual cycles of the wife are necessary for following up her basal body temperatures. During this time separate interviews are held with husband and wife and all problems involved in AID are thoroughly discussed. In the first place we try to verify the level and the stability of their emotional relations and to test the real desire for a child. At the same time, both the prospects and the dangers of AID are pointed out. The personal contact with the married couple and the evaluation of their personality are, in our opinion, of paramount importance in the period previous to the procedure. A written agreement by both husband and wife to the treatment requested by them is an obvious prerequisite of AID.

TABLE 1

SEMINOLOGICAL FINDINGS IN 219 MEN, WHOSE WIVES WERE TREATED BY THERAPEUTIC DONOR INSEMINA-TION

Seminological findings	No. of cases
Azoospermia	143
Severe oligozoospermia	57
Oligo-asthenospermia	19
Total	219

Before starting treatment a routine gynaecological investigation is performed. The estimation of the appropriate time for AID is made on the basis of basal temperature records. Fresh semen from healthy men with normal seminological values were always used for treatment. The number of spermatozoa was always higher than 40 million/ml, their motility was mostly good or fair and the percentage of morphologically defective forms did not exceed 30%. In the insemination procedure about 0·5 ml of semen was introduced into the first part of the cervical canal and the remainder was deposited in the posterior fornix. The patient was then left for 30 min on the examination table with the pelvis elevated. In most cases only a single insemination was performed in the course of each menstrual cycle.

RESULTS

Among a total of 219 patients inseminated, 132 conceptions were obtained in 114 women. These results achieved in the 'successful' subgroup are summarized in Table 2.

Additional information concerning Table 2 is as follows: from three twin pregnancies there were five live children and one macerated still-born foetus. One male foetus died *intra partum* owing to compression of the umbilical cord. Two male foetuses died within 10 days after delivery: one died 10 hr after delivery by Caesarian section at the 8th month because of placenta praevia; the other one died on Day 7 following normal delivery, the cause of death being unknown.

In analysing the duration of 109 pregnancies we found that most deliveries (ninety-one cases) occurred between the 38th and the 42nd week of pregnancy. There were two post-mature pregnancies (over 42 weeks) and in sixteen women birth took place before the 38th week. Of these, three foetuses were immature, between the 33rd and 36th week. There was one developmental anomaly, a boy with penile hypospadias.

TABLE 2

RESULTS OF 132 PREGNANCIES FOLLOWING AID

Total number of pregnancies	132	
Births including three sets of twins		109
Living boys		50, about 46%
Living girls		58, about 54%
Death during delivery		1
Death within 10 days after delivery		2
Spontaneous abortions		14
Pregnancies in an advanced stage		8
Result unknown		1
Total	132	

TABLE 3

DATA ON THE NUMBER OF MENSTRUAL CYCLES OF AID NEEDED FOR 131 CONCEPTIONS IN 104 PATIENTS

Menstrual cycle in which AID was successful	Deliveries or advanced pregnancies		Abortions	
	No.	%	No.	%
1	40	34·2	6	43·0
2	18	15·4	2	14·3
3	16	13·7	2	14·3
4	13	11·1	1	7·1
5	11	9·4	1	7·1
6	6	5·1	–	–
7	4	3·4	1	7·1
8	4	3·4	–	–
9	3	2·5	–	–
10	1	0·9	1	7·1
15	1	0·9	–	–
Total	117	100·0	14	100·0

Table 3 gives the data on the number of inseminations needed for 117 pregnancies through AID. One hundred and nine of them went to term and in eight cases the patients were in an advanced stage of pregnancy at the time of reporting. The second column indicates corresponding data on fourteen spontaneous abortions.

In the 'successful' subgroup consisting of 114 women, 503 therapeutic inseminations resulted in 132 conceptions. The mean number of inseminations/conception was 3·8.

One hundred and five patients out of a total of 219 failed to conceive; these constitute the 'unsuccessful' subgroup, and Table 4 records the menstrual cycle in which these patients terminated treatment.

15

In the 'unsuccessful' subgroup, 601 inseminations were performed in the 105 women, which corresponds to a mean rate of 5·7/one patient.

Complications following the treatment by AID, such as losses during pregnancy and delivery, have already been mentioned in Table 2, as well as the developmental anomaly of one male child. In one case vaginal trichomoniasis appeared after insemination. Two patients divorced. The wife of a hypogonadotrophic eunuchoid, who had a child by AID, was unhappy 2 years later and complained of the very low sexual activity of her husband; the latter, however, refused treatment for this defect.

TABLE 4

DATA ON THE TERMINATION OF TREATMENT BY THERAPEUTIC DONOR INSEMINATION IN THE 'UNSUCCESSFUL' SUBGROUP

Cycle, in which the treatment by AID was terminated	Cases	
	No.	%
1	16	15·2
2	25	23·8
3	17	16·2
4	8	7·7
5	8	7·7
6	7	6·6
7	5	4·8
8	5	4·8
9	1	0·9
10	3	2·8
Over 10	10	9·5
Total	105	100·0

Out of ten patients in whom more than ten AID were carried out, one was inseminated 24 times, one 47 times, the remaining eight between 11 and 20 times.

DISCUSSION

Of 219 women treated by AID over the course of 15 years we obtained 132 conceptions in 114 patients. This 'successful' subgroup constitutes about 52% of the total number. When evaluating the number of conceptions in relation to the total number of the women who were treated (132 conceptions in 219 women) we reach the 60·2% level, which corresponds quite well with the results achieved by other authors (see Behrman, 1959).

Comparing the 'successful' and the 'unsuccessful' subgroups, we found that patients unsuccessfully treated by AID were more frequently older (over 30 years of age), that the percentage of regular menstrual cycles was significantly lower in them and that their gynaecological findings offered a distinctly lower chance of success in AID than in patients constituting the 'successful' subgroup. We are fully aware that a more critical selection of women patients would increase the percentage of successful results by AID and let us approach the 75% level (Haman, 1954; Behrman, 1959). However, we sometimes deliberately performed therapeutic donor insemination for 'psychological' reasons in patients in whom the chances of success were known to be poor. The analysis of data on the number of inseminations (see Table 4) shows that in the 'unsuccessful' subgroup the women patients often terminated the treatment prematurely (after inseminations in two or three menstrual cycles only). This may be because both husband and wife feel a certain degree of psychic relaxation arising from a conviction that, in their endeavour to cure the sterility of their marriage, they have exhausted all the therapeutic possibilities.

In the 'successful' subgroup (see Table 3) we found that, in nearly 90% of cases, conception occurred in the course of six menstrual cycles. In most cases, therefore, we consider the therapeutic possibilities of AID to be practically exhausted, if insemination is performed for five to six menstrual periods. Because of this experience we complete the gynaecological investigation by hysterosalpingography or endometrial biopsy only when AID performed throughout five or six cycles has remained unsuccessful and when the married couple wishes the treatment to be continued. In the 'successful' subgroup the mean rate of therapeutic trials per conception was comparatively low at 3·8.

The evaluation of our results as to losses in pregnancy shows their rate to be approximately the same as in conceptions following normal sexual intercourse (seventeen losses in 132 conceptions, that is nearly 13%). Only two patients out of twelve gave up AID because of losses in pregnancy; the remaining ten continued or are continuing it, and eight of them have already given birth to children.

A full knowledge of both husband and wife, a careful evaluation of their emotional attitudes and mutual relations, and the development of a feeling of mutual trust require at least several months and are perhaps the most important prerequisite for AID. For these reasons therapeutic donor insemination can never become a current medical procedure in widespread use. In our experience, if we are to proceed cautiously, we find we are able to carry out this treatment for only fifteen to twenty married couples at a time. About eight to ten women are likely to conceive in the course of 1 year.

In this way it will be possible to reduce the number of unavoidable complications to the lowest possible figure. As opposed to the few cases where complications occur, there are large numbers of marriages where therapeutic donor insemination consolidates married life and makes it fuller. In our 'successful' subgroup twenty-two patients out of 114 requested further insemination after the birth of the first child. We are of the opinion that, in married couples afflicted by sterility, with happy emotional relations and normal gynaecological findings, AID is a very effective form of treatment which contributes to strengthening the family and to enhancing marital happiness.

REFERENCES

BEHRMAN, S. J. (1959) Artificial insemination. *Fert. Steril.* 10, 248.
BEUERLEIN, I. (1963) *Die künstliche Samenübertragung beim Menschen im angloamerikanischen Bereich.* Beiträge zur Sexualforschung, 29. Heft. Ferd. Enke Verlag, Stuttgart.
HAMAN, J. O. (1954) Results in artificial insemination. *J. Urol.* 72, 557.
KLEEGMAN, S. J. (1954) Therapeutic donor insemination. *Fert. Steril.* 5,
SCHELLEN, A. M. C. M. (1957) *Artificial insemination in the human.* Elsevier Publishing Company, Amsterdam.

17

Frozen human semen for artificial insemination

GEORGE W. MATHESON, M.D.

LARS CARLBORG, M.D.

CARL GEMZELL, M.D.

FREEZING OF human sperm for insemination has several advantages. Ejaculates can be collected at a time when qualified donors are available and used at a later time as needed without having the donor available on demand. Matching of donor and recipient can be more selective as a wide variety of donor somatic characteristics and blood groups can be made readily available with the use of a sperm bank. Freezing the semen of an oligospermic husband provides material for pooling and insemination of his wife at the time of ovulation.

Early attempts at freezing semen by Jahnel,[8] Shettles,[18] Hoagland and Pincus,[6] and Parkes[10] resulted in recovery of a small number of viable sperm. In 1949 Polge,

Smith, and Parkes[12] described the advantages of using glycerol as a protective agent for sperm during freezing. Sperm freezing has been widely utilized in the field of dairy husbandry, but experience with human spermatozoa freezing and storage has been limited. In 1953 Sherman and Bunge[16] described the successful freezing at $-70°$ C. in dry ice and subsequent recovery of human sperm. In later reports, the same group eventually recorded 9 pregnancies in 26 patients.[3, 4, 9] In 1963 Sherman[17] described a freezing method using liquid nitrogen with a storage temperature of $-196°$ C. Using this method Perloff, Steinberger, and Sherman[11] reported 6 pregnancies and later Steinberger and Perloff[19] reported 13 pregnancies, although in neither report was the total number of patients or inseminations noted.

Sawada and co-workers[7, 13, 14] used a rapid freezing method with dry ice and obtained 10 pregnancies in 150 patients treated. Using the same dilution media (7.5 per cent

This investigation was supported in part by Public Health Service Fellowship 1-F2-HD-31,545-01 from the National Institute of Child Health and Human Development.

18

glycerol in egg yolk–citrate) but freezing in liquid nitrogen and controlling the rate of cooling to match an experimentally determined slower pattern,[14] Behrman and Sawada[2] in 1966 reported 14 pregnancies in 28 patients. Although previous methods showed good motility recovery, this was the first time that there was a definitely successful method as measured by a high percentage of pregnancies. In fact, it was noted that there was a poor correlation between the motility recovery and the ability of the thawed semen to fertilize. In order to freeze the semen with this method it was necessary to use an expensive controlled rate freezing apparatus. Sawada and Ackerman[15] suggested replacing this controlled-rate freezer with alcohol baths but did not report any results with this modification.

A method has now been devised to successfully freeze human sperm with the use of basic equipment commonly found in most hospital laboratories. The purpose of this report is to describe in detail this simplified technique of human sperm freezing and handling. In addition, its use in providing frozen donor sperm for successful patient insemination is described.

Material and methods

Collection and examination. Semen specimens were obtained by ejaculation and allowed to liquify. An aliquot was removed for routine analysis, including motility, concentration, and morphology. No ejaculate was used for donor insemination if the initial motility was less than 50 per cent, the concentration was less than 60 million per milliliter, or morphologic examination showed greater than 30 per cent abnormal forms. In addition, sperm penetration evaluation was performed according to the method described by Carlborg, McCormick, and Gemzell.[5] Cervical mucus was obtained from fertile donor women in midcycle. It was frozen and stored in micro–hematocrit capillary tubes at –4° C. After thawing the mucus, a drop of sperm was placed at one end of the tube in connection with the mucus. The distance of fartherest sperm penetration was microscopically observed in 5 minutes. Penetration greater than 2.0 mm. at this time was considered adequate. A total of 54 semen samples from 10 donors was frozen, thawed, and evaluated.

Preparation of protective media. The protective media used were a modification of that described by Behrman and Sawada.[2] The media mixture consists of egg yolk, 20 per cent by volume; glycerol, 15 per cent by volume; 5.5 per cent glucose in water, 26 per cent by volume; and 3 per cent sodium citrate in water, 39 per cent by volume. To each milliliter of the final solution a mixture of glycine 15 mg. and erythromycin 1 mg. was added. The resultant mixture was warmed in a water bath at 56° C. for 30 minutes and then cooled to room temperature. The pH was adjusted to 7.2-7.4 with 1.4 per cent sodium bicarbonate solution. If more than 10 per cent of the total media volume of this solution was needed to correct the pH, a 0.1N sodium hydroxide solution was used to complete the pH correction. The media were then stored in tightly stoppered amber glass bottles at +4° C. for as long as 3 months.

Freezing. The ejaculate was then mixed with this protective media in 1:1 ratio at room temperature by adding the media dropwise to the semen, while gently agitating the latter. After mixing the semen with the media, a 10 to 15 minute equilibration period was allowed. The semen media mixture was then drawn into 0.5 ml. cylindrical 130 mm. × 3 mm. plastic straws.* The ends of the straws were sealed with a moisture solidifying powder* (Fig. 1). From each ejaculate 8 to 12 straws were usually obtained.

Five or six straws were then placed into a standard 13 cm. glass test tube with 1 mm. walls containing 95 per cent ethyl alcohol at room temperature. The alcohol level was sufficient to cover the semen media mixture in the straws. The tubes containing the straws were cooled for 25 minutes at 4° C. with occasional agitation. The tubes were then transferred to a beaker containing 95 per

*Societe Anonyme, Instruments de Medecine Veterinaire, L'Aigle, France.

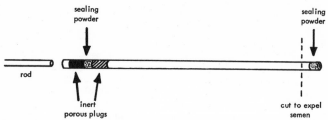

Fig. 1. Plastic straws used for freezing and storage of semen-media mixture. The rod is used to expel the sample after cutting the end from the tube.

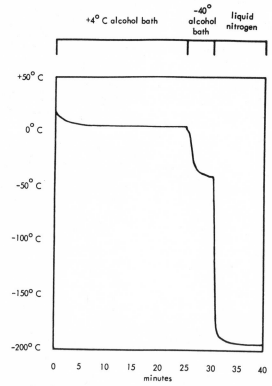

Fig. 2. Representation of the temperature changes within a sample of semen during cooling.

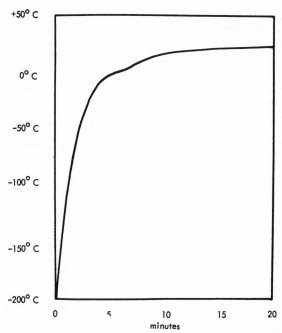

Fig. 3. Representation of the temperature changes within a sample of semen during thawing in air at room temperature.

cent ethyl alcohol which was stored at –40° C. in an electric freezer. The levels of alcohol in the test tubes and the bath were equal. After 5 minutes in the –40° C. bath, the straws were rapidly transferred to a Linde LR-35 liquid nitrogen freezer* and cooled to and stored at –196° C.

This method of cooling was evolved by modifying a general pattern of freezing previously found to be advantageous, using pregnancies as the criteria of success.[2, 15] A thermocouple was placed into a straw filled with the semen media mixture and the pattern of cooling took place as follows: From room temperature to 4° C. at an average rate of slightly less than 1° C. per minute; 4° C. to –30° C. at an average of 7° C. per minute, and then rapidly to –196° C. in the liquid nitrogen (Fig. 2).

*Union Carbide Corporation, Linde Division, New York.

Thawing. The semen media specimens were thawed in air at room temperature (Fig. 3). A temperature of +20° C. was reached in 12 to 14 minutes. The samples were observed for motility and penetration and comparison made to the values before freezing as a mesaure of recovery.

Clinical application

The frozen sperm was used for donor artificial insemination in 7 selected infertility couples who were found to be infertile, primarily on the basis of oligospermia or azoospermia of the husband. The women were seen daily beginning 4 days prior to expected ovulation, as determined by history of past cycles. Basal body temperature, the physical characteristics of the cervix and cervical mucus, and karyopyknotic index were noted daily. In addition, a sample of the recipient's cervical mucus was obtained daily and tested for sperm penetrability. One straw of semen media was thawed and one drop used for both motility evaluation of the sperm as well as the in vitro Carlborg penetration test. This procedure allowed a direct physiologic evaluation of both the donor sperm and the patient's receptivity to it. If penetration was adequate (greater than 2.0 mm. per 5 minutes), the remainder of the semen in the straw was used for that day's insemination by placing it directly into the patient's lower cervical canal. A control straw from each ejaculate was always evaluated against known receptive mucus before the ejaculate was designated for donor use. If penetration on the daily in vitro testing between donor and recipient was inadequate, the sperm was tested with known receptive mucus to ascertain whether the failure was due to the recipient mucus or the donor thawed semen sample. If the problem was due to the thawed semen sample, another frozen sample was utilized. When in vitro penetration was good and insemination was started, in vitro penetration testing was carried out daily until the penetration rate dropped, indicating ovulation had occurred in the recipient. At this time inseminations were stopped. In no case was insemination continued more than a total of 4 days.

The semen media mixture can be directly expelled from the straw into the endocervical canal or into the endometrial cavity, by exerting gentle pressure with a small metal rod applied to the plugged end after the sealer is amputated (Fig. 1). All successful inseminations in this report were performed at the external os.

Results

The semen motility recovery rate is defined as $\dfrac{\%\text{ motility after thawing}}{\%\text{ motility before freezing}} \times 100$.
The mean semen motility recovery rate in the 54 samples from 10 donors used to evaluate the method prior to clinical use was 58 per cent. All samples tested showed 80 per cent or greater of their initial penetration when known receptive cervical mu-

Table I. Effect of delay in initiation of cooling on postthaw recovery*

Time from ejaculation to start of cooling (hr.)	Mean postthaw motility (%)	Mean motility recovery rate (%)
<1	31	48
1- 3	21	29
3- 6	14	21
6-12	6	11

*Each figure is based on one ejaculate from each of 8 donors. Samples from one ejaculate underwent initiation of cooling at varying intervals following collection and mixing with media.

Table II. Evaluation of thawing technique*

Method of thawing	Mean postthaw motility (%)	Mean motility recovery rate (%)
37° C. water bath	18	27
Air at room temperature	35	51
4° C. water bath	26	40

*Each figure is based on one ejaculate from each of 10 donors. Samples for each ejaculate were thawed simultaneously under each condition.

cus was used both prior to freezing and after thawing. Thawing for motility evaluation was generally carried out one day following freezing. Re-evaluation of these samples during storage up to 180 days showed no further significant decrease in motility.

When several samples from a single ejaculate mixed with media were cooled at varying time intervals after collection, the time delay was found to adversely affect the postthaw motility recovery rate. A drop in recovery was noted if initiation of cooling was delayed greater than one hour following ejaculation (Table I). There was a constant initial loss of 10 to 20 per cent in motility when the semen samples were mixed with the media but not frozen. When this mixture was left at room temperature, there was noted little further loss in motility over a 6 hour period.

The motility recovery rate was determined to be lower when thawing was performed in water baths at 37° C. or 4° C. instead of at room temperature (Table II).

To date seven patients have been treated for at least one cycle by the method of evaluation and insemination outlined. Three patients became pregnant, 2 during the first and one during the second cycle of treatment. Of those who have not yet conceived, 2 have been treated for one cycle, one for two cycles, and one for four cycles. The donor inseminations in these patients were performed with semen obtained from 6 donors. Samples had been stored up to 83 days. Correlation between motility recovery rate and pregnancy was poor. Donor ejaculate used in the successful conceptions had a sperm motility recovery rate of 35 to 50 per cent. In these specimens the absolute postthaw motility varied from 25 to 45 per cent. Postthaw semen-mucus penetration rates were in the acceptable range in all successful inseminations. They were also adequate in most cycles in which conception did not occur. All pregnancies ended in normal deliveries at term.

Comment

A simple, reasonably economical method has been developed for the handling, freezing, and utilizing of frozen human semen. The present work demonstrates a simplification of freezing schedules already found to be effective.[2, 15] The use of readily available and reasonably inexpensive equipment permits the application of this method to centers not engaged in major research undertakings in the field. The liquid nitrogen freezer is the only special device needed and may be obtained at a moderate cost.

Prompt handling and adequate evaluation of each ejaculate appear to be necessary to obtain adequate semen recovery rates. Delay in initiation of freezing resulted in decreased recovery rates which were found to be unrelated to prolonged contact with media in the unfrozen state.

Introduction of the straw as a container for the human semen media mixture offers a number of advantages. The small volume in each straw allows a large number of separate samples to be obtained from each ejaculate. Each one of these samples is sufficient for successful insemination. This separation provides enough samples for adequate in vitro testing of each ejaculate after thawing as well as material for two or more courses of insemination. By use of the straw as the instrument for insemination, additional handling of the semen is eliminated. Because of the small volume and large surface area within the straw, the semen media mixture is cooled more evenly throughout.

Timing the insemination remains a formidable problem in any attempt in this field. By using the straws, an adequate small amount of semen from the same ejaculate can be delivered to the cervix (or higher if necessary) over a several-day period. The use of one sample a day for many days may offer the best chance of success in patients who ovulate at irregular intervals. The use of the straws provides the necessary means of extending the ejaculate over this long period.

By testing the ability of a given sample of thawed sperm to penetrate the recipient's cervical mucus at the time of intended insemination and then using that sample of semen for insemination, it is felt that a more physiologic evaluation is made of the patient's receptivity. Although the other standard methods of ovulation detection were employed, the Carlborg penetration test seemed most useful. From this simple test the physician can gain much insight into the viability of the sperm, the physical and hormonal condition of the patient's reproductive system, and the interaction of the semen and female reproductive tract at their first point of contact. Further analysis of the clinical results and correlation with in vitro studies must await a more lengthy application of the method.

Although the use of this method for insemination with the husband's semen has been attempted only once to date, it is hoped to further these studies. Semen of males with oligospermia could be collected, stored, centrifuged, and then pooled for a concentrated insemination at the time of his wife's ovulation. The husband's sperm can be frozen for use if he is unable to be present when the woman ovulates, such as during FSH treatment at a remote center. Still another application is the male who is impotent but can periodically deliver an ejaculation by masturbation.

Of the small number of patients treated, 43 per cent are pregnant. Of the patients who are pregnant a mean of only 1.4 inseminations were required as opposed to 2.8 by Behrman and Sawada[2] using frozen semen and 3.5 when using fresh donor sperm.[1] Although the clinical evaluation of this method is still preliminary, the results are encouraging.

REFERENCES

1. Behrman, S. J.: Internat. J. Fertil. **6:** 291, 1961.
2. Behrman, S. J., and Sawada, Y.: Fertil. & Steril. **17:** 457, 1966.
3. Bunge, R. G., Keettel, W. C., and Sherman, J. K.: Fertil. & Steril. **5:** 520, 1954.
4. Bunge, R. G., and Sherman, J. K.: Nature **172:** 767, 1953.
5. Carlborg, L., McCormick, W., and Gemzell, C.: Acta endocrinol. **59:** 636, 1968.
6. Hoagland, H., and Pincus, G.: J. Gen. Physiol. **25:** 337, 1942.
7. Iizuka, R., and Sawada, Y.: Jap. J. Fertil. **3:** 1, 1958.
8. Jahnel, F.: Klin. Wchnschr. **17:** 1273, 1938.
9. Keettel, W. C., Bunge, R. G., Bradbury, J. T., and Nelson, W. O.: J. A. M. A. **160:** 102, 1956.
10. Parkes, A. S.: Brit. M. J. **2:** 212, 1945.
11. Perloff, W. H., Steinberger, E., and Sherman, J. K.: Fertil. & Steril. **15:** 501, 1964.
12. Polge, C., Smith, A. U., and Parkes, A. S.: Nature **164:** 666, 1949.
13. Sawada, Y.: Jap. J. Fertil. **4:** 1, 1959.
14. Sawada, Y.: Internat. J. Fertil. **9:** 525, 1964.
15. Sawada, Y., and Ackerman, D. R.: *In* Behrman, S. J., and Kistner, R. W., editors: Progress in Infertility, Boston, Little, Brown & Company. In press.
16. Sherman, J. K., and Bunge, R. C.: Proc. Soc. Exper. Biol. & Med. **82:** 686, 1953.
17. Sherman, J. K.: Fertil. & Steril. **14:** 49, 1963.
18. Shettles, L. B.: Am. J. Physiol. **128:** 408, 1940.
19. Steinberger, E., and Perloff, W. H.: AM. J. OBST. & GYNEC. **92:** 577, 1965.

ARTIFICIAL INSEMINATION

William J. Curran, LL.M., S.M.Hyg.

ARTIFICIAL insemination has been a practice in human beings and in animal species for a very long time. It is mentioned in the *Talmud* and other ancient writings.[1] Yet it took until 1968 for the highest court of an American state to face and to decide the important legal issues presented by heterologous [third-party donor] artificial insemination. In *People v. Sorensen*,[2] the Supreme Court of California decided in a unanimous opinion that a child conceived by AID to a married woman with the knowledge and consent of her husband is the legitimate offspring of the marriage.

The facts of the case were not in dispute and were as follows: the couple had been married for 15 years and were childless. It was medically determined that the husband was sterile. The couple consulted a physician in San Francisco and both consented to the artificial insemination. They signed an agreement on the letterhead of the doctor requesting the procedure. The semen was to be selected by the physician and under no circumstance was the couple to be told the name of the donor. A male child was born to the wife in 1960. The information for the birth certificate was supplied by the wife and it named the husband as the father. The defendant father said he had not seen the birth certificate until this trial for nonsupport.

For some four years the couple lived together and the child was treated as and was represented to friends as the child of the couple. In 1964, the mother left her husband and took the child with her. At the time of the separation, the mother told the husband she wanted no support for the child and she consented to a divorce being granted the husband. After an illness, in 1966, she was unable to work and sought public assistance. It was after this that the support order was obtained against the husband.

The Supreme Court upheld the conviction of the husband and specifically declared that he was, under the facts, the "lawful father" of the child. It was held that this term is not limited to the biological or natural father. The determining factor, said the court, is whether a legal relationship of father and son exists. It was found that it does. It was noted that the anonymous donor could not be considered the natural father "as he is no more responsible for the use made of his sperm than is the donor of blood or a kidney."

The California Court also refused to rule AID to be an adulterous act. Under California law, the argument that the act was criminal adultery was found "absurd."

The *Sorensen* case probably will not end the controversy over artificial insemination; there are still too many religious, moral, and social conflicts surrounding it. However, the case should help to settle the legal issues raised concerning the procedure. Most of the doubt cast upon AID has appeared in the "scare literature" of some popular medical periodicals which seem to revel in arousing legal fears in their medical readers. On the contrary, it should be pointed out that not one American state has a statutory prohibition of artificial insemination. One American state, Oklahoma, in 1967 specifically authorized it under statutory procedures and declared such a child to be legitimate.[3] Therefore, the procedure of artificial insemination, under the traditional rules of American criminal jurisprudence, must be deemed lawful in all states. Furthermore, no American court of highest jurisdiction has found AID to be adulterous. There is no recorded case of even an attempt to prosecute a person involved in AID for the crime of adultery, let alone a conviction for such a "crime."

An intermediate appellate court in New York held in 1963 that an AID child conceived with the husband's consent was illegitimate, but that the husband was nevertheless liable for the support of the child.[4] However, in the same case the court annulled the marriage on other grounds as never consummated, thus making the case distinguishable from the Sorensen case, where the marriage relationship was fully valid.

A Canadian decision, *Orford v. Orford*,[5] decided in 1921, is often cited as holding an AID procedure adulterous. However, in this case, the wife was inseminated *six years after separation* from her husband and without his consent or knowledge. In court she explained her action on the grounds that the "treatment," which resulted in a child, was intended to cure her dyspareunia (abnormally painful intercourse). The Canadian Court had little sympathy for her and allowed the husband a divorce on the grounds of adultery. A Scottish court came to the opposite conclusion in 1958, holding AID even without the husband's consent was *not* adultery and *not* grounds for a divorce.[6]

American physicians, using AID and wishing to assure the legality of the procedure and the legitimacy of any offspring, would be wise to follow the practices outlined in the *Sorensen* case. They should require evidence that the couple is validly married, that the marriage is not subject to annulment, and that the couple is then living together. The records of the physician should contain documents signed by both wife and husband, requesting and consenting to the procedure and agreeing to raise any resulting child as their own. For the protection of the physician, the agreement should stipulate that the physician alone will select the donor and semen, that the name of the donor will not be disclosed to the couple, and that the physician does not guarantee that conception of a child or that a normal child will necessarily result from the procedure.

Some practitioners in the field advise against the use of written records in order to protect privacy and to prevent later use of the records to prove that the husband did not sire the child. These are commendable reasons. However, the *Sorensen* case shows the value of written records as proof of the knowledge, consent, and participation of the husband in the procedure. These records, which can be otherwise kept confidential, eventually protected the *child*, which should be the first concern of the physician in all cases.

REFERENCES

1. Kardimon, Artificial Insemination in the Talmud, *Hebrew Med. J.*, 2:164 (1950).
2. 66 Cal. Rptr. 7, 437 P.2d 495 (1968).
3. Oklahoma Annotated Laws, Title 10, §§551–553. See also New York City Health Code, Art. 21 (1959).
4. *Gursky v. Gursky*, 39 Misc. 2d 1083, 242 N.Y.S. 2d 406 (1963).
5. 58 D.L.R. 251 (1921).
6. *Maclennan v. Maclennan*, [1958] Sess. cas. 105, [1958] Scots L.T.R. 12.

**Artificial Insemination in Cattle
and Horses**

MOTION PICTURE ANALYSIS OF EJACULATION IN THE BULL

G. E. SEIDEL, Jr AND R. H. FOOTE

INTRODUCTION

Recent evidence indicates that sperm losses in the artificial vagina (AV) for bulls amount to 12 to 14% of the ejaculate (Foote & Heath, 1963; Seidel, 1968). These losses may be related to the pattern of semen emission in the AV. Bonadonna (1956) observed that emission normally occurred at the time of maximum extension of the penis. This study was initiated to obtain more information about the pattern of ejaculation in normal bulls.

MATERIALS AND METHODS

Semen was collected from eight 3-year-old Holstein-Friesian bulls at weekly intervals for 7 weeks. One ejaculate was collected per bull during the 1st week and two successive ejaculates were taken at 50-min intervals on each collection day thereafter. During the first 5 weeks, a 30-cm AV coupled to a 45-cm lucite extension tube was used at a temperature of 55° C. During the 6th and 7th weeks, this AV at 55° C and a 15-cm AV with the lucite extension at 40° C were used. The two AVs were used consecutively and in both orders for first and second ejaculates. After the 1st week of semen collection, 16-mm colour motion pictures were taken of the penis through the transparent lucite tube. Ektachrome type B film was used at 64 frames per second (fps). During the 4th week, motion pictures were taken of the entire bull during semen collection at 24 fps.

Data obtained during Weeks 3, 4 and 5 were subjected to the analysis of variance assuming a complete factorial design comprised of the factors: bulls, weeks, and successive ejaculates. Ejaculate volume, sperm concentration, and initial progressive motility of spermatozoa were determined for each ejaculate. The following criteria were estimated by examining the film with a viewer or dissecting microscope: (1) the length of the penis extension from the AV entrance; (2) the stimulus time, defined as the time elapsing from contact of the penis with the AV until the emission of semen began, (3) the actual semen emission time, and (4) the degree of coiling of the penis. Criteria 2 and 3 were determined by counting the number of frames between events, and multiplying by the frame time of 1/64 sec. The degree of coiling of the penis was assigned numerical values as described in Table 1.

Intense sexual preparation was maintained throughout the experiment. A padded steel dummy was used exclusively for the collection of semen from one of the bulls, and similar collections were made from several of the other bulls during the first few weeks.

RESULTS AND DISCUSSION

Means for Weeks 3 to 5 are presented in Table 1. The AV at 55° C was used for semen collections during this period. The average values for the ejaculates were a volume of 6·4 ml, a sperm concentration of $1·58 \times 10^9$ spermatozoa/ml and an initial motility of 58%. Bull differences in length of penis extension were not large $(P<0·1)$, but were substantial considering that bulls were of similar age (33 to 41 months). Bull differences are likely to be greater in the general population, indicating the desirability of providing AVs of appropriate length for different bulls. Bulls also differed in stimulus time $(P<0·05)$ and the amount of coiling of the penis $(P<0·005)$. There was more coiling with first than with second ejaculates $(P<0·05)$. Subjectively, the coiling appeared to be associated with the more vigorous thrusts. All bulls showed coiling to some extent (Table 1), suggesting it is a normal occurrence. Coiling previously recorded (Carroll, Ball & Scott, 1963; Ashdown & Coombs, 1967) was usually observed before mating or during electro-ejaculation and, under these conditions, may have been an abnormality.

An increase in length of penis extension and semen emission time occurred in the course of the experimental period and means of 8·2, 9·9 and $10·9 \times 10^9$ total spermatozoa per ejaculate for Weeks 3, 4 and 5, respectively, also reflect an increase, suggesting a more effective removal of spermatozoa from the epididymis. These increases may have resulted from incomplete adjustment to the experimental regimen, although the first 2 weeks' data were discarded.

Significant $(P<0·05)$ correlation coefficients obtained were $r = -0·33$ between stimulus time and ejaculate volume, $r = -0·30$ between stimulus time and total spermatozoa per ejaculate, and $r = -0·30$ between stimulus time and length of penis extension. Since a long stimulus time represented a slow thrust, these correlations suggest that improper preparation or stimulation leads to a less vigorous thrust and fewer spermatozoa per ejaculate.

From the data obtained, an approximate diagram of the position and rate of movement of the tip of the penis during a typical ejaculation was prepared (Text-fig. 1). Semen emission normally occurred when the penis was fully extended or slightly earlier. The relative position and rate of movement of the penis just before the thrust, and especially after emission, depended in part upon the collection technique. Ejaculations with the AV at 55° C did not involve multiple thrusts or emissions. However, many of the ejaculations using the AV at 40° C did not fit the normal pattern of Text-fig. 1. Evaluation of these was more subjective and, therefore, trends rather than numerical values are presented for Weeks 6 and 7.

TABLE 1

MEANS OF MAIN EFFECTS

Factor	Factor level	Length of penis extension (cm)	Stimulus time (sec)	Semen emission time (sec)	Frequency distribution of coiling[d]				Mean coiling[e]
					0	1	2	3	
Weeks	3	49·9[a]	1·05	0·26[b]	8	3	1	4	1·06
	4	54·3	1·00	0·30	9	2	3	2	0·88
	5	56·0	0·85	0·32	6	1	6	3	1·38
Ejaculates	1	54·8	0·90	0·30	8	3	6	7	1·50[b]
	2	52·0	1·06	0·29	15	3	4	2	0·71
Bulls	1	59·5[c]	1·03[b]	0·29	2	1	0	3	1·67[a]
	2	49·9	1·23	0·33	3	0	2	1	1·17
	3	50·6	0·98	0·31	2	1	1	2	1·50
	4	52·7	1·28	0·30	5	0	1	0	0·33
	5	54·9	0·83	0·28	2	0	2	2	1·67
	6	53·8	0·86	0·27	1	1	3	1	1·67
	7	55·3	0·55	0·30	5	0	1	0	0·33
	8	50·4	0·87	0·27	3	3	0	0	0·50
Grand mean or total		53·4	0·97	0·29	23	6	10	9	1·10

[a] = Statistical significance within the array, $P < 0.005$; [b] $P < 0.05$; [c] $P < 0.10$. [d] 0 = no coiling; 1 = slight coiling; 2 = moderate coiling; 3 = extensive coiling ($\sim 360°$). [e] = Non-parametric techniques were used for statistical tests of coiling.

Greater coiling of the penis appeared to be positively related to the length of penis extension and negatively related to stimulus time. There was much less coiling associated with the shorter AV at the lower temperature used in sequence with the standard AV during Weeks 6 and 7. This low level stimulus treatment also resulted in slightly less extension of the penis and a longer semen emission time. With this treatment, semen emission sometimes lasted longer than a second and often there were multiple emissions. Such ejaculates were high in volume and low in sperm concentration. The penis was often extended and retracted several times.

Plate 1 depicts a coiling sequence enlarged from the motion pictures of semen ejaculation. Emission of semen continued for a number of frames beyond

Pl. 1, Fig. 3 and lasted for 0·29 sec. If the sequence shown in Pl. 1 is taken as representing maximum coiling, the amount of coiling shown in Pl. 1, Fig. 2 would be coded as 2 and that shown in Pl. 1, Fig. 3 as 3 (Table 1). The coil was retained, in part, for a total of 0·51 sec. The pattern and duration of coiling and the relationship between coiling, semen emission and maximum penis extension varied with ejaculates. An ejaculate without coiling of the penis appeared essentially as an extension of Pl. 1, Fig. 1.

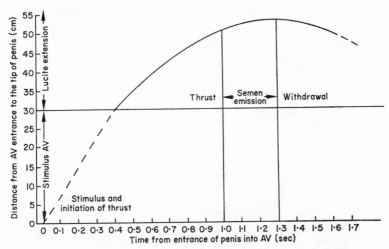

TEXT-FIG. 1. Time–motion study of approximate movements of the penis during semen collection with an artificial vagina (AV). The solid line represents observations made through the lucite extension of the AV and the dashed lines represent extrapolations. The ordinate is an indication of penis extension.

The potential semen loss from spermatozoa adhering to the side of the AV is shown well in Pl. 1, Figs. 2 and 3. Much of this loss could be avoided with a shorter AV which would allow emission to occur nearer the collecting cone, though the optimum length of AV would vary for individual bulls (Table 1). It appears that the photographic method can be used to determine this optimum for any set of conditions.

A rhythmic wiggling of the fore-limb dew claws was observed in the motion pictures during semen collection. These dew claws represent vestigial second and fifth digits. The significance of this phenomenon is unclear; it may be associated with sexual excitement.

The study of feet and leg movements during Week 4 showed both rear feet leaving the ground during thrusting in thirteen of fifteen collections and one rear foot left the ground in the other two cases. In this behaviour pattern, the bulls studied appeared to be normal (Hafs, Knisely & Desjardins, 1962).

Additional features can best be observed in the motion picture film. A 7-min 16-mm colour film was prepared highlighting several of the features seen in the experimental film (Seidel & Foote, 1967).

31

PLATE 1

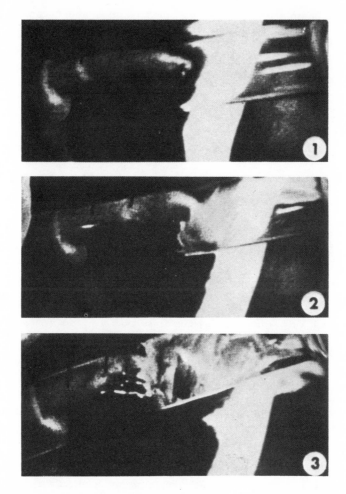

Sequence showing ejaculation in the bull, omitting several of the consecutive frames. Lines on the artificial vagina (AV) were 5 cm apart.

FIG. 1. This picture, showing the first drop of semen emitted, was taken approximately 0·45 sec after the initiation of thrust into the AV.

FIG. 2. Formation of the coil photographed approximately 0·06 sec after Fig. 1.

FIG. 3. Complete coiling of the penis approximately 0·19 sec after Fig. 1.

ACKNOWLEDGMENTS

Bulls and collection facilities were provided by Eastern A.I. Cooperative, Inc. and photography was by Morris Brock.

REFERENCES

ASHDOWN, R. R. & COOMBS, M. A. (1967) Spiral deviation of the bovine penis. *Vet. Rec.* **80,** 738.

BONADONNA, T. (1956) Sull' uso corretto della vagina artificiale ed azione riflessa nel comportamento sessuale del *Bos taurus*. *Veterinaria ital.* **7,** 885.

CARROLL, E. J., BALL, L. & SCOTT, J. A. (1963) Breeding soundness in bulls. A summary of 10,940 examinations. *J. Am. vet. med. Ass.* **142,** 1105.

FOOTE, R. H. & HEATH, A. (1963) Effect of sperm losses in semen collection equipment on estimated sperm output by bulls. *J. Dairy Sci.* **46,** 242.

HAFS, H. D., KNISELY, R. C. & DESJARDINS, C. (1962) Sperm output of dairy bulls with varying degrees of sexual preparation. *J. Dairy Sci.* **45,** 788.

SEIDEL, G. E., JR (1968) *Effect of collection interval and artificial vagina length and temperature on the bovine ejaculate, compartmental analysis using biochemical markers, and motion picture analysis of ejaculation.* M.S. thesis, Cornell University.

SEIDEL, G. E., JR & FOOTE, R. H. (1967) *Ejaculation in the bull* (a motion picture). Department of Animal Science, Cornell University.

AN IMMUNE RESPONSE TO EGG-YOLK SEMEN DILUENT IN DAIRY COWS

J. F. T. GRIFFIN, W. R. NUNN AND P. J. HARTIGAN

INTRODUCTION

Since Landsteiner (1899) first discovered the antigenic properties of bovine spermatozoa, antibodies to the semen of mice (McLaren, 1964; Edwards, 1964; Bell, 1969a), rabbits (Edwards, 1960; Behrman & Nakayama, 1965; Menge, 1968; Bell, 1969b), guinea-pigs (Isojima, Graham & Graham, 1959; Katsh, 1959) and cattle (Menge, 1967) have been found following iso-immunization of the female with semen or testis. The antigenicity of semen varies from species to species and while guinea-pigs (Isojima *et al.*, 1959) and cattle (Menge, 1967) give a good immunological response, prolonged iso-immunization in the presence of adjuvants is necessary to induce antibodies in mice (McLaren, 1964) and rabbits (Edwards, 1960). Even with cattle, however, chemical adjuvants must be incorporated with the semen or no immunological reaction is found (Kiddy, Stone, Tyler & Casida, 1959). Fertility is reduced in females showing high serum titres of antibody to homologous spermatozoa following iso-immunization (Katsh, 1959; McLaren, 1964; Behrman & Nakayama, 1965; Menge, 1967).

Serum titres of sperm agglutinating antibodies have been demonstrated in cattle following repeated service (Bratanov & Dikov, 1959; Sokolovskaja & Reshetnikova, 1968) and in women with a history of unexplained infertility (Franklin & Dukes, 1964; Tyler, Tyler & Denny, 1967). However, the work of Menge (1967) has shown that natural service of cattle does not elicit an immune response, even in animals presensitized with homologous semen before service.

With artificial insemination (AI) in cattle, the bovine genital tract is exposed not only to iso-antigenic semen but also to highly antigenic proteins such as egg-yolk and skimmed milk, which are routinely used in solution as diluents for the semen. Bratanov, Dikov & Popova (1962) have demonstrated serum titres of antibody to egg-yolk semen diluent in heifers inseminated early in the *postpartum* period with semen diluted in egg-yolk diluent. Subsequently, they observed an allergic response and missed fertilization, when these animals were inseminated with semen diluted in the same diluent.

In this report, serological tests on serum, tissue and mucus samples from the genital tracts of cows receiving repeated inseminations, showed that, although antibody titres to egg-yolk diluent were isolated from the majority of samples, no significant immune response was found to homologous seminal antigens.

MATERIALS AND METHODS

In a preliminary study, uterine mucus and biopsy samples were collected repeatedly from 104 dairy cows, all of which were impregnated by AI. Samples were taken after insemination and never later than 10 days following service. Animals which had not been inseminated nor served naturally were used as controls. In a second group of sixty-eight cows, all of which were artificially inseminated, samples were taken simultaneously from the vagina, uterus and serum on a single occasion. Ten cows served naturally were used as controls.

Biopsy samples were obtained from the vagina and uterus using an instrument designed by Hartigan, Murphy & Nunn (unpublished data). Mucus was obtained with this instrument and with cotton wool swabs introduced into the tract by the technique used for microbiological sampling (Murphy, 1967). All samples were transferred to 2-ml amounts of physiological saline and stored at 4° C. Tissue samples were homogenized with a ground-glass pestle and mortar and centrifuged to remove cellular débris. The mucus was solubilized with glass beads on a vibrator (Fisons) before centrifugation. Blood was collected from the jugular vein and the serum decanted after clotting. All test samples were heated at 56° C for 30 min and stored at −19° C.

The AI station responsible for the insemination of the test animals supplied samples of fresh bovine semen which had been stored at 4° C, and also samples of semen which had been diluted in egg-yolk diluent and stored at 4° C or deep frozen in liquid nitrogen. All semen samples were washed five times in Krebs' buffered saline (Wales, Martin & O'Shea, 1967) before use in the agglutination tests. Seminal plasma was obtained by centrifuging the semen samples at 2500 rev/min for 10 min. Lactose egg-yolk diluent (Nagassi) was used for the dilution of semen and the tests *in vitro*.

A modification of the passive haemagglutination test of Boyden (1951) was used to detect antibodies to seminal plasma and egg-yolk diluent. Human (ORh+) red blood cells, preserved by treatment with formalin (Weir, 1967), were treated with tannic acid before coating with the test antigen. Haemagglutination inhibition tests were carried out using soluble antigen, in order to confirm the specificity of the reaction. Untreated 'tanned' cells and negative sera were used as controls. Sperm agglutination tests were carried out using the microscopic technique of Kiddy et al. (1959) and the macroscopic agglutination-in-gel reaction of Kilbrick, Balding & Merrill (1952). In the sperm immobilization test (Ashitaka, Isojima & Ukita, 1964), human serum was used as a source of complement. Negative sera and saline were used as controls in all tests.

In all immunological tests, titres of less than 16 were found with the control samples, so that only titres greater than this were regarded as positive.

RESULTS

In the preliminary study, antibodies to egg-yolk diluent were demonstrated frequently in the homogenates of uterine mucus and biopsy samples taken from the 104 dairy cows. The frequency with which positive titres were found rose concomitantly with the number of services the animal had received before collection of the sample (Table 1). Antibody titres to egg-yolk diluent were

TABLE 1

THE CORRELATION BETWEEN THE INCIDENCE OF UTERINE ANTIBODY TITRES TO EGG-YOLK DILUENT AND THE FREQUENCY OF SERVICE

	No. of services		
	0	1 to 3	≥4
No. of animals tested	20	40	49
No. showing titres	1	15	37
% showing titres	5	37·5	77·5

found in the uterine samples from the majority of animals served four or more times (repeat-breeders).

The antibody titres found in the uterine samples ranged from 64 to 256, with the higher titres occurring in the animals with the greater number of services.

Samples from eighty of these animals were examined for antibodies to spermatozoa and seminal plasma. Of these, two animals which had been served five and seven times, gave titres of 32 and 64, respectively.

To determine the site of origin of the antibody found in the uterus, samples taken simultaneously from the vagina, uterus and serum of sixty-eight cows were examined. Only tests for antibody to egg-yolk diluent were carried out.

The frequency with which positive titres were obtained from these samples is given in Table 2. These results show that the vagina was the site from which antibodies were isolated most frequently, while the lowest immunological response was found in the serum samples.

Although antibodies were shown to be present in the vagina and uterus of many of these cows, the source of these antibodies was not known. A correlation between the titres found in the serum and vagina of a selected group of animals is given in Table 3. This shows that, of twenty-three animals which had positive titres in the vagina, nineteen had positive serum titres. Of these nineteen animals, ten had vaginal titres greater than those found in the serum.

Four animals had vaginal titres in the absence of any humoral response so that of twenty-three animals which had vaginal titres, fourteen had titres which could not be accounted for entirely by the passage of humoral antibody into the tissues of the genital tract. This can be explained by the production of local antibody by the vagina following exposure to diluent antigens.

TABLE 2

RELATIONSHIP BETWEEN ANTIBODIES TO EGG-YOLK
DILUENT AND FREQUENCY OF SERVICE BY AI

	No. of services by AI before testing		
	0*	1 to 3	≥4
Serum positive	0/10	12/25	18/31
% positive	0	48	58
Vaginal biopsy positive	0/7	10/14	13/15
% positive	0	71·5	86·7
Uterine biopsy positive	1/6	7/12	8/12
% positive	16·7	58·4	66·7

* This includes animals served naturally, which had not been brought into contact with semen diluent at service.

TABLE 3

CORRELATION BETWEEN VAGINAL AND SERUM TITRES OF ANTIBODY
TO EGG-YOLK DILUENT ANTIGENS

	Vagina+	Vagina+ Serum+	Vagina+ Serum−	Vagina− Serum+
No. of animals with antibody titres to egg-yolk diluent	23	19	4	2

A similar comparison was made between uterine and serum titres. Although the antibody titres found in uterine homogenates were lower than those in the vagina, they were also found both in excess and in the absence of serum titres.

Tests were carried out *in vitro* to determine the effect of these antibodies on semen homologous to that used in the service. Fresh semen and semen which had been diluted and stored in egg-yolk diluent was washed and tested for sperm agglutination and immobilization. Samples which had titres to diluent antigens in the passive haemagglutination test caused mixed agglutination of the spermatozoa which had been stored in egg-yolk diluent but did not have any effect on the semen which was stored and diluted in saline, except for causing non-specific head-to-head agglutination. Immobilization of spermatozoa was not demonstrated using spermatozoa stored in egg-yolk diluent or saline.

The fertility of forty animals from which samples had been obtained follow-ing the first, second or third service was examined in order to evaluate the effect of antibodies to the egg-yolk diluent. The fertility of fifteen animals which had uterine titres following a given service was significantly lower ($P \geqslant 0.05$) than the fertility of twenty-five animals in which there were no uterine titres (Table 4).

TABLE 4

THE ASSOCIATION BETWEEN UTERINE ANTIBODIES TO EGG-YOLK DILUENT AND FERTILITY

| | Uterine titres to diluent antigen | |
	+	−
No. of animals	15	25
No. repeating to the service following which the sample was obtained	14	13
% repeating to the service	93·4%*	52%*

* Differences significant at $P \geqslant 0.05$.

Uterine titres of antibody to semen were found so infrequently that they could not be associated with the reduced breeding efficiency.

DISCUSSION

Although Bratanov & Dikov (1959) and Sokolovskaja & Reshetnikova (1968) have found antibodies to homologous spermatozoa in the serum of cattle following service, it would appear that semen provides a weak immunological challenge to cattle under these conditions. Chemical adjuvants must be used in conjunction with homologous semen to induce antibodies in cattle under experi-mental conditions (Kiddy et al., 1959; Menge, 1967). Bratanov, Dikov, Radev & Danov (1965, 1966) have found increased titres of iso-antibodies to sperma-tozoa following service of animals suffering from such diseases as latent chronic endometritis or oestrual metrorrhagia, and they suggest that there may be an accelerated absorption of spermatozoa which induces serum titres of antibody with greater facility than in normal animals.

Bratanov et al. (1965, 1966) did not attempt to assess the antifertility effect of the humoral iso-antibodies to semen nor did they establish the significance of such antibodies within the genital tract. Menge (1967) found that, following iso-immunization of heifers with semen, antibody titres could be found con-currently in the serum and the uterus, and that there was a direct correlation between the level of titres in the uterus and the breeding efficiency of the host. The extremely low incidence of uterine titres to homologous semen (2·5%), found in the present work, would suggest that under natural conditions, high titres of antibodies to semen are not frequently produced even in animals served repeatedly.

In contrast to this, antibodies to egg-yolk semen diluent antigens were frequently detected in the vagina, uterus and serum of cattle after repeated service by AI. Our results would suggest that these antibodies may be produced locally in the genital tract of cattle and/or in the humoral system, following service. The important factor is that, irrespective of the site of production, the antibodies may be present within the genital tract and therefore could affect the fertility of the female.

The different agglutination patterns obtained *in vitro* on testing homologous spermatozoa which had been stored in egg-yolk diluent or saline, with samples which had titres to diluent protein, would suggest that storage of spermatozoa in egg-yolk diluent alters their antigenicity. Under natural conditions, seminal-plasma antigens become attached to the mammalian sperm surface as the spermatozoa pass through the male genital tract (Weil & Rodenburg, 1962). The negatively charged surface of the bovine sperm surface (Veres & Oscenyi, 1968) would provide an optimal environment for the ionic binding of protein molecules, such as egg-yolk diluent protein. Such a reaction could cause occlusion of the normal antigenic sites of the spermatozoa and confer on them an antigenicity similar to diluent protein, thus making them sensitive to agglutination by antibody specific for egg-yolk diluent antigen. Bratanov, Dikov & Tornjov (1968) have found similar types of agglutination patterns with the immune serum from rabbits immunized with bovine semen diluted in egg-yolk diluent. Swanson & Hunter (1969) have demonstrated clumping when rabbit spermatozoa, which had been diluted in egg-yolk diluent, were mixed with specific antisera for the egg-yolk diluent antigen. No agglutination or immobilization could be demonstrated with the antisera.

A reduction in fertility of animals to service with semen diluted in egg-yolk diluent was found in the present work, when uterine titres to diluent antigens were present, as compared with animals showing no titres. From these results, it would appear that the presence of antibodies to egg-yolk diluent in the bovine uterus, is detrimental to the fertility of AI service. Swanson & Hunter (1969) have shown that rabbit antisera to egg-yolk semen diluent alone does not reduce the fertility of semen stored in homologous diluent, when used to treat the semen before insemination. They propose that the presence of these antibodies within the tissues of the uterus may interfere with fertility.

Preliminary results have shown that the fertility of rabbits to insemination with semen diluted in egg-yolk diluent was significantly reduced in animals which had high titres of antibody to diluent antigen. Ten of eleven rabbits which had uterine mucus titres of less than 64 were fertile following insemination, whereas none of seven animals with mucus titres equal to or greater than 64 was fertile. Although a direct correlation was found between antibodies to egg-yolk diluent and infertility, no relationship could be found between reduced fertility and uterine titres to seminal antigens (Griffin, McGilligan, Hartigan & Nunn, in preparation). From our results, it would appear, therefore, that the presence of antibodies to semen diluent antigens in the uterus of cows or rabbits can have an adverse effect on the breeding performance.

ACKNOWLEDGMENTS

We wish to thank the Agricultural Institute, Chemical Services Ltd, and the Ballyclough and Galtee Cattle Breeding Stations for their financial support and the provision of technical facilities.

We are also grateful to Professor J. T. Baxter for his interest in this work.

REFERENCES

Ashitaka, Y., Isojima, S. & Ukita, H. (1964) Mechanism of experimental sterility induced in guinea pigs by injection of homologous testis and sperm. II. Relationship between sterility and a sperm-immobilizing antibody. *Fert. Steril.* **15**, 213.

Behrman, S. J. & Nakayama, M. (1965) Antitestis antibody: its inhibition of pregnancy. *Fert. Steril.* **16**, 37.

Bell, E. B. (1969a) Immunological control of fertility in the mouse: a comparison of systemic and intravaginal immunization. *J. Reprod. Fert.* **18**, 183.

Bell, E. B. (1969b) Iso-antibody formation against rabbit spermatozoa and its effect on fertility. *J. Reprod. Fert.* **20**, 519.

Boyden, S. V. (1951) The adsorption of proteins on erythrocytes treated with tannic acid and subsequent haemagglutination with antiprotein sera. *J. exp. Med.* **93**, 107.

Bratanov, K. & Dikov, V. (1959) Investigations on spermoisoagglutination in connection with the fertilization of cows. *Nauchni Trud. nauchno-izled. Inst. Razvad. Bol. izskustv. Osemen. selskostop. Zivotn. (Sofija)*, **1**, 11. *Anim. Breed. Abstr.* **30**, No. 965.

Bratanov, K., Dikov, V. & Popova, J. (1962) On some agglutination phenomena of bovine spermatozoa when diluted in egg-yolk and preserved with antibiotics. *Akad. na Selsk. Nauk. Sofia Nauchno-izsled. Inst. po Biol. i Patol. na Razmnozhavaneto na Selsk. Zhivotni Izv.* **3**, 11.

Bratanov, K., Dikov, V., Radev, G. & Danov, D. (1965) Investigations on the immunology of reproduction. VII. On the role of spermoantibodies in the insemination of cows with incomplete involution of the uterus and cows having latent endometritis. *Vet. Sci.* **2**, 323.

Bratanov, K., Dikov, V., Radev, G. & Danov, D. (1966) Investigations on the immunology of reproduction. VIII. On the role of spermoantibodies in repeated insemination of cows having oestral metrorrhagia. *Nauchni Trud. vissh selskostop. Inst. Georgi Dimitrov,* **16**, 333.

Bratanov, K., Dikov, V. & Tornjov, A. (1968) Sur la spécificité des antigènes de spermatozoïdes dans le sperme du taureau. *VIe Congr. Int. Reprod. Anim. Insem. Artif., Paris,* **1**, 529.

Edwards, R. G. (1960) Antigenicity of rabbit semen, bull semen and egg yolk after intravaginal or intramuscular injections into female rabbits. *J. Reprod. Fert.* **1**, 385.

Edwards, R. G. (1964) Immunological control of fertility in female mice. *Nature, Lond.* **203**, 50.

Franklin, R. R. & Dukes, C. D. (1964) Antispermatozoal antibody and unexplained infertility. *Am. J. Obstet. Gynec.* **89**, 6.

Isojima, S., Graham, R. J. & Graham, J. B. (1959) Sterility in female guinea pigs induced by injection with testis. *Science, N.Y.* **129**, 44.

Katsh, S. (1959) Infertility in female guinea pigs induced by injection of homologous sperm. *Am. J. Obstet. Gynec.* **78**, 276.

Kiddy, C. A., Stone, W. H., Tyler, W. T. & Casida, L. E. (1959) Immunological studies on fertility and sterility. III. Effect of isoimmunization with blood and semen on fertility in cattle. *J. Dairy Sci.* **42**, 110.

Kilbrick, S., Balding, D. L. & Merrill, B. (1952) Methods for detection of antibodies against mammalian spermatozoa. II. Gelatin agglutination technique. *Fert. Steril.* **3**, 430.

Landsteiner, K. (1899) Zur Kenntnis der spezifisch auf Blutkorperchen wirkenden Sera. *Zentbl. Bakt. Parasitkde,* **25**, 546.

McLaren, A. (1964) Immunological control of fertility in female mice. *Nature, Lond.* **201**, 582.

Menge, A. C. (1967) Induced infertility in cattle by iso-immunization with semen and testis. *J. Reprod. Fert.* **13**, 445.

Menge, A. C. (1968) Fertilization, embryo and fetal survival rates in rabbits isoimmunized with semen, testis and conceptus. *Proc. Soc. exp. Biol. Med.* **127**, 1271.

Murphy, J. A. (1967) *An investigation into the microbiology of the genital tract of normal and repeat-breeding dairy cows in Ireland.* Ph.D. thesis, Dublin University.

Sokolovskaja, I. I. & Reshetnikova, N. M. (1968) Immunological factors in fertilization and early embryonic development. *Zhivotnovodstvo, Mosk.* **6**, 65.

Swanson, L. V. & Hunter, A. G. (1969) Egg-yolk antigens and their effect on fertility in rabbits. *Biol. Reprod.* **1**, 324.

Tyler, A., Tyler, E. T. & Denny, P. C. (1967) Concepts and experiments in immunoreproduction. *Fert. Steril.* **18**, 153.

Veres, I. & Oscenyi, A. (1968) Recent results obtained from ultrastructural examination of bull sperm cells. *VIe Congr. Int. Reprod. Anim. Insem. Artif., Paris,* **1**, 213.

Wales, R. G., Martin, L. & O'Shea, T. (1967) Effect of dilution rate and number of spermatozoa inseminated on the fertility of rabbits ovulated with chorionic gonadotrophin. *J. Reprod. Fert.* **10**, 69.

Weil, A. J. & Rodenburg, J. M. (1962) The seminal vesicle as a source of the spermatozoa coating antigen of seminal plasma. *Proc. Soc. exp. Biol. Med.* **109**, 567.

Weir, D. M. (1967) *Handbook of experimental immunology.* Blackwell Scientific Publications, Oxford.

40

Semen Placement Effects on Fertility in Bovines

J. W. MACPHERSON

A number of investigators have compared fertility levels resulting from semen placement at various sites in the reproductive tract of the cow using the rectovaginal technique (1-4). However, some doubts as to the actual location of placement must exist due to recent observations, indicating that technical accuracy can be as low as 25% (5). In addition, it has been extremely difficult to have sufficient numbers of animals inseminated to split portions of an ejaculate before the advent of frozen semen.

This study was undertaken to accurately measure the effects of semen placement at three depths to simulate mid-cervical, deep cervical or os uteri, and intrauterine deposition.

Experimental Procedures

One ejaculate was collected from each of nine bulls, three located at each of three artificial insemination cooperatives. Semen was extended in sterile milk extender containing penicillin and streptomycin (6). The final glycerol concentration was 10% by volume. Semen samples contained at least 70% motile spermatozoa initially and were extended to contain 50×10^6 motile spermatozoa per milliliter of extender before freezing in glass ampules and storing in liquid nitrogen.

Regular plastic insemination rods were equipped with plastic discs 1.5 cm in diameter cemented to the rods at distances of 4, 8, and 12 cm from the tip. The discs were colored white, red, and black, respectively, and the inseminators instructed to record on the breeding slip the disc color used for the insemination. A mean total of 51 ± 5.4 first inseminations was made to each ejaculate at each depth. In all cases inseminations were first breedings. The insemination rods were selected at random, inserted into the cervical opening, and moved anteriorly as far as the disc would permit, at which time 1 ml of extended semen was expelled. All inseminations were done during a 30-day period. Fertility results were calculated on a 60- to 90-day nonreturn basis.

Results and Discussion

A summary of the over-all fertility results appears in Table 1. Analysis of variance indicated that there were no significant bull differences. Significant differences between treatments were observed. Duncan's new multiple-range test (9) indicated that the fertility rate obtained following semen placement at the 8-cm depth was significantly better ($P < .05$) than that obtained with semen placed at the 4-cm depth. This finding is not in agreement

41

TABLE 1. Field fertility results comparing semen placement at three locations in the bovine.

Description	Mean fertility level	SD
Placement 4 cm anterior to the external uterine orifice	63.15	±8.52
Placement 8 cm anterior to the external uterine orifice	73.56	±4.16
Placement 12 cm anterior to the external uterine orifice	68.21	±8.38

Experimental error degrees of freedom, 16; error mean square, 43.18.

with observations of others (6). However, it has been demonstrated that accuracy of semen placement is questionable without some device to control the site of deposition (5).

The depths selected for semen deposition were chosen to represent semen placement intracervically at 4 cm, uterine body at 8 cm, and uterine horn at 12 cm in young but sexually mature animals (7). However, in some older cows the 4- and 8-cm depths could both be considered as intracervical depositions (8).

Under conditions of this experiment it would appear that maximum fertility results can be anticipated when deep cervical or uterine body sites are selected for semen placement. These findings agree with the general practices of cattle insemination techniques in Canada and the United States. It is recommended when cervical insemination in bovines is practiced that the application be deep within this organ.

Acknowledgment

The financial assistance of the National Research Council of Canada Grant no. A-2378 was appreciated.

References

(1) Drennan, W. G., and J. W. Macpherson. 1966. The reproductive tract of bovine slaughter heifers. Canadian J. Comp. Med. Vet. Sci., 30: 224.
(2) King, G. J., and J. W. Macpherson. 1965. Observations on retraining of artificial insemination technicians and its importance in maintaining efficiency. Canadian Vet. J., 6: 83.
(3) Knight, C. W., T. E. Patrick, H. W. Anderson, and C. Branton. 1951. The relation of site of semen deposit to breeding efficiency of dairy cattle. J. Dairy Sci., 34: 199.
(4) Macpherson, J. W. 1960. Sterile milk as a semen diluent. Canadian Vet. J., 1: 551.
(5) Olds, D., D. M. Seath, M. C. Carpenter, and H. L. Lucas. 1953. Interrelationships between site of deposition, dosage, and number of spermatozoa in diluted semen and fertility of dairy cows inseminated artificially.

J. Dairy Sci., 36: 1031.

(6) Patrick, T. E., and H. A. Herman. 1953. Missouri University Agr. Exp. Sta., Res. Bull. 526.

(7) Salisbury, G. W., and N. L. VanDemark. 1951. The effect of cervical, uterine, and cornual insemination on fertility of the dairy cow. J. Dairy Sci., 34: 68.

(8) Sission, S., and J. D. Grossman. 1940. The Anatomy of Domestic Animals. 3rd ed. Saunders Co., New York, N.Y.

(9) Steel, G. D., and J. H. Torrie. 1960. Principles and Procedures of Statistics. McGraw-Hill Inc., New York.

The use of A.I. Centre Records in Applied Science

J. P. FRAPPELL M.R.C.V.S

THE primary objectives of an A.I. service are the attainment of pregnancies by the use of semen from superior males. An efficient A.I. service has a two-fold effect—firstly, that of putting the female, without delay, into an economically viable productive state (*e.g.* the dairy cow into milk, the sow with litter) and, secondly, that of creating a generation which is a little better, genetically speaking, than the dam. One could also mention, as a third effect, that if, as is usual, only first inseminatons are chargeable and repeat inseminations are free, its own finances benefit.

For an A.I. service to determine the individual outcome, in terms of confirmed pregnancies, of large numbers of inseminations a year would be a time-consuming and expensive process. It is possible, however, to arrive at a closely correlated situation by recording all inseminations, both first and repeat, and calculating the percentage of females which receive first inseminations but receive no second insemination within a given period of time after the first. Provided that numbers in the sample are adequate, this " non-return " percentage is a reliable yardstick for comparing efficiencies of techniques, individual bulls, and inseminators and the fertility of different female groups or populations.

44

The following phenomena and situations have been studied to determine their effect, if any, on non-return rates and fertility. A number of these situations arise in assessments veterinary surgeons have to make during day-to-day work in cattle practice.

Seasonal effects.
Herd size
Breed.
Calving to service interval.
Newly established herds.
Natural Service v. A.I.

As previously stated, it is not usual for A.I. centres to obtain data on the final outcome of all inseminations. However, occasions and needs arise when it is necessary or informative to determine the outcome of pregnancies and to record data on parturition, calves, etc. Calving difficulties and peri-natal survival are of particular significance in the context of the assessment of certain cross-breeding programmes and also in the evaluation of the progeny test data for individual dairy bulls. Both factors are also of immediate and long-term consequence to the individual farmer.

Surveys of calf losses made in A.I. herds and also in herds covered by M.M.B. Business Costings Services are reviewed.

Data obtained in the investigation of the results of Charolais inseminations has produced additional information on calf birthweights, gestation periods and regional differences in these values.

The detection of bulls that may be carrying genes for abnormal anatomical or physiological features is a major responsibility associated with animal breeding. To control the propagation of possibly undesirable features, it is important to know the frequency of occurrence of such features within the breed population. An effective centralised reporting system is a pre-requisite for proper control, and such a system is operated at the Board's Head Office.

Some of the data collected through these routine monitoring systems and also through special surveys and analyses, are presented in the following histograms, graphs and tables—together with a brief introduction to the subject matter.

45

Providing that number of inseminations included are large enough to rule out chance effects it is possible to predict quite accurately, from the 30/60 day non-return percentage, the percentage figures at the 60/90 and 90/120 day intervals. The 30/60 day figure may be used as a reliable measure of efficiency of individual units, bulls and inseminators. (See histogram below.)

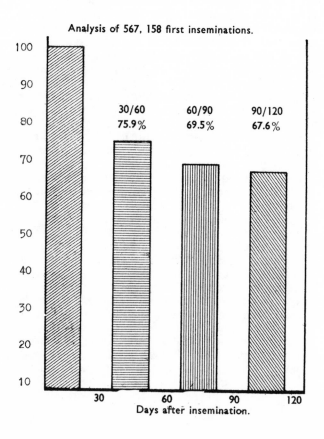

Analysis of 567, 158 first inseminations.

Table I shows the depression in N.R. rates that normally arises when a group of cows are inseminated at a single visit. This is not due to any fall in inseminator efficiency but is due to one or more cows in the group being mistakenly observed as showing signs of true oestrus behaviour. This is the principal cause of the apparently lower fertility level in the larger herd when this level is assessed purely on a non-return rate basis.

TABLE I

No. of Animals Inseminated at One Visit
Effect on N.R. Per Cent. (2,466 Cows 1963)

No. of cows	N.R. per cent.
2	72·5
3	66·6
4	67·0
5	56·5

Both surveys (see graph on right) show a decline in non-return percentage as numbers of cows in the herd increase —at least to the 120 cow herd size. This decline in N.R. percentage does not necessarily mean the herd is less fertile —it would, in part at least, be due to an increased proportion of cows being put forward for insemination when not in heat, etc. (see Table I).

A considerable amount of data, from studies conducted in many countries, shows that the chance of successful conception and pregnancy increases as the interval between calving and insemination lengthens. This rise in fertility has to be offset against the most economic calving interval (normally taken as 365 days) in determining when the cow should receive her first post-calving insemination. If this insemination takes place after the 60 day interval it is normally possible to fit in up to two inseminations, if necessary, and still have the cow calving at about the 12 month interval.

The E. Region survey shows that almost 20 per cent. of cows are given a first insemination within 52 days of calving. Seventy per cent. of cows receive a first insemination before reaching their maximum fertility level.

47

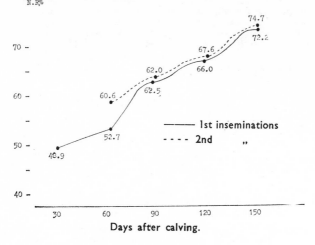

Welsh Region 1950 2,647 cows.

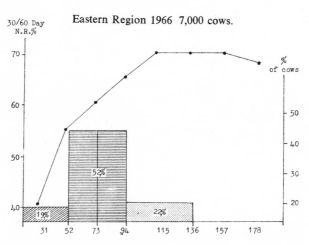

Eastern Region 1966 7,000 cows.

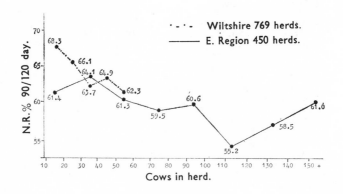

48

In each of the three years, January and May have the lowest N.R. percentage rate at the 30/60 day interval. Contrary to what is often believed, April and May are certainly not months of high fertility. The second half of the year has a higher overall non-return rate than the first half of the year. (See histograms on right.)

TABLE II
BREED OF COW. EFFECT ON N.R. PER CENT.
(1966 E. Region 450 Herds)

No. of services	Percentage holding to service	
	Friesians	Others
1	62·4 ⎱ 84·2	59·3 ⎱ 82·4
2	21·8 ⎰	23·1 ⎰
3	9·2	9·8
4	3·7	4·1
5	1·6	1·8
6	1·3	1·9
Average No. of services per assumed conception	1·64	1·72

Table II (above) shows the Friesian cow as being marginally superior to cows of other breeds in respect of fertility—as judged by non-return rates. One factor that must not be ignored, however, is the possible tendency to allow the dairy cow of a breed other than Friesian further "repeat" inseminations because of her lower slaughter value as a cull cow.

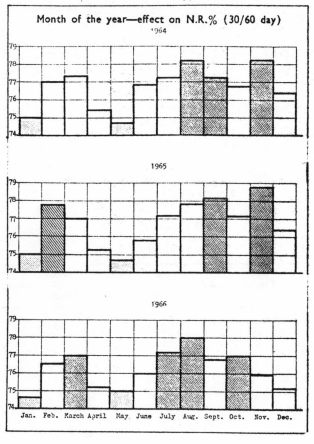

Month of the year—effect on N.R.% (30/60 day)

1964

1965

1966

50

Table III (below). These figures show the factual position achieved during a 12 month period. Well in excess of 95 per cent. of the inseminations would have been carried out with unfrozen semen. In the case of some breeds, e.g. Devon, Aberdeen Angus and Hereford, most of the insemination would have been on cows of a different breed. Strictly comparable selection pressures would not have operated in the case of each breed in respect of bull fertility —the dairy breeds would have been carrying a greater proportion of older " proven " sires, for example.

TABLE III
BREED OF BULL. EFFECT ON N.R. PER CENT.
(National Year 1963/1964 30/60 day)

Breed	First inseminations '000	N.R. Per cent.
Welsh Black	13	81·2
Galloway	6	79·6
Devon	45	78·5
Aberdeen Angus	180	78·4
Dairy Shorthorn	34	77·1
Friesian	713	77·0
Hereford	446	77·0
South Devon	4	75·0
Sussex	12	74·7
Ayrshire	101	73·3
Guernsey	78	72·8
Jersey	61	72·8

Breeds with less than 5,000 first inseminations excluded.

TABLE IV
EFFECT OF HERD ESTABLISHMENT TIME
(Welsh Region 1958 789 herds. 6,231 cows)

Period 1958	125 New herds		664 Other herds	
	Cows	N.R. per cent.	Cows	N.R. per cent. (90/120 day)
1st quarter	364	61·2	1,626	70·8
2nd quarter	251	55·7	1,372	72·3
3rd quarter	141	69·5	1,001	75·7
4th quarter	165	60·0	1,311	78·6
Year	921	60·8	5,310	73·7

Table IV (above). Changing individual cows to a new environment, through their transfer to another herd, appears to cause a depressed fertility level for at least 12 months following transfer. The Welsh Region study was made in herds restocked after foot-and-mouth disease in 1957/58. Further studies of a similar nature will be made in herds restocked after the 1967/68 outbreaks.

51

Tables V, VI, VII, VIII, and IX (below and right) compare fertility levels in herds using A.I. and Natural Service. The controversy over the relative efficiency of the two methods has existed since commercial A.I. services began operating and will presumably continue for some time to come. Comparisons can be based on one or more of the various ways of assessing fertility levels—e.g. non-return rates, services per conception, herd calving intervals, percentage of dry cows. The herds in Table V were chosen in advance of the year over which records were assembled, purely on their willingness to co-operate in collection of the information. Tables VI and IX are based on pairs of herds matched in terms of size, breed and other management factors.

TABLE V
CONCEPTION AND CALVING RATES
COMPARISON OF NATURAL SERVICE AND A.I. HERDS
(3 Regions 1966 4,392 cows)

Herd category		A.I.	N.S.
No. of herds		59	35
No. of cows		3,443	1,489
Conception rate	1st	61·6	65·8
	1st + 2nd	81·1	83·6
Barren rate		6·9	8·6
Live calving rate		89·9	86·7

Conception rate differences at 1st—not significant
                    at 1st + 2nd—not significant
Live calving rate difference   —just significant

TABLE VI
CALVING INTERVALS
NATURAL SERVICE HERDS AND A.I. HERDS
200 N.M.R. HERDS 1966

Type of service	Average calving interval
Only natural service	395 days
Only A.I.	387 days

Difference of eight days highly significant.

TABLE VII
CALVING INTERVALS AYRSHIRE BREED
NATURAL SERVICE HERDS AND A.I. HERDS

Herd average calving interval: (days)	A.I. herds	Non-A.I. herds
	Per cent. of herds in group	
Less than 370	6·0	10·8
370–379	14·5	13·3
380–389	20·5	19·3
390–399	30·1	28·9
400–409	18·1	13·3
410–419	6·0	8·4
420–429	2·4	4·8
Over 429	2·4	1·2

Acknowledgments to Livestock Record Bureau—Edinburgh.

TABLE VIII
CALVING INTERVALS AYRSHIRE BREED
NATURAL SERVICE HERDS AND A.I. HERDS

	1959		1960	
	A.I. herds	Non-A.I. herds	A.I. herds	Non-A.I. herds
No. of herds	39	39	44	44
Cows per herd	41	50	46	54
Yield (gallons)	847	822	858	822
Fat per cent.	3·82	3·82	3·82	3·82
Calving intervals (days)	392	392	394	393

Acknowledgments to Livestock Record Bureau—Edinburgh.

TABLE IX
PERFORMANCE OF L.C.P. HERDS USING
NATURAL SERVICE ONLY
AND A.I. ONLY

Physical factors	Natural service	A.I.
Milk yield per cow (gallons)	764	814
Concentrate use (lb. per gallon)	2·7	2·7
Average percentage of dry cows	21·2	19·4
Average number of cows per herd	58	53

50 herds in each group 1966.

The data in Table X (below) arises from an analysis of records maintained by members of a Farm Costings Service (Low Cost Production) operated by the M.M.B. for milk producers.

TABLE X
CALF MORTALITY
Calves born dead or dying within seven days of birth

(L.C.P. data 1963. 353 herds. 17,430 calvings)

Breed of dam				Total calvings	Per cent. mortality
Friesian	...	...	...	7,863	6·9
Ayrshire	...	...	...	3,931	4·5
Guernsey	...	...	...	695	10·6
Jersey	...	...	...	976	7·6
Mixed	...	...	...	3,965	5·5
Total ...		...	...	17,430	6·2

The data in Table XI (below) was obtained by all inseminators in the organisation, who were operating on a specific day in each month, seeking the answers to a set of questions at farm visits where a responsible person was available.

TABLE XI
CALF LOSSES IN A.I. HERDS
(Monthly survey June 1963-May 1964)

Average No. of herds surveyed each month					...		2,050
Average No. of calves up to eight weeks old on day of visit	...	...	...	...	...	...	6,159
Average annual loss rate (from birth to eight weeks)							
Homebred calves	...	...	...	...	...		6·3%
Heifers	...	...	...	...	...	4·1	
Bulls	...	...	...	...	...	8·0	
Purchased calves	...	...	...	...	...		13·5%

TABLE XII
SEX RATIO OF CALVES
EFFECT OF AGE OF SIRE (4,315 calvings 1960)

	No.	Average Age	Total calves	Per cent. male	Per cent. female
Old bulls	32	11·1	1,908	50·16	49·84
Young bulls	39	3·0	2,407	49·56	50·44
				Difference not significant	

Table XII (above) shows the result of an investigation made to determine whether there was any substance in the belief that younger bulls sired a higher proportion of female calves than did older bulls. There was no significant difference between the two age groups.

TABLE XIII
BIRTHWEIGHT OF CALVES FROM FRIESIAN COWS
BY SIRES OF THREE DIFFERENT BREEDS

Region	Sire		
	Charolais	Hereford	Friesian
North	96·42	88·81	90·27
Wales	102·70	85·15	84·56
Midland	101·04	90·33	89·92
South East	100·36	90·10	86·81
South West	107·87	95·75	93·55
Average	101·67	90·02	88·98

Birthweights corrected to standard gestation period of 283·6 days. Each extra day calf is carried it gains 0·65 lb ± 0·012 lb. Charolais Report 1966.

Tables XIII and XIV (above and below). Following the first importation of Charolais bulls to the U.K. in November, 1961, and their subsequent A.I. use, a large amount of data became available on birthweights of various breeds of calves.

One unexpected outcome was the variation in average birthweight of calves between different geographical regions of England and Wales.

A subsequent trial in which Friesian bulls only were used showed that a significant difference existed between Regions and that this was not due to individual bulls.

TABLE XIV
DEVIATIONS OF MEAN BIRTHWEIGHT FROM
THE BREED AVERAGE—REGIONAL EFFECT

Region	Breed of sire		
	Charolais	Hereford	Pure-bred
North	—5·21 lbs	—1·22 lbs	+1·29 lbs
Wales	+0·86 ,,	—4·87 ,,	—4·42 ,,
Midlands	—0·59 ,,	+0·29 ,,	+0·94 ,,
South East	—1·27 ,,	+0·07 ,,	—2·37 ,,
South West	+6·21 ,,	+5·73 ,,	+4·56 ,,

Charolais Report 1966.

A Modified Equine Artificial Vagina for the Collection of Gel-Free Semen

John C. Ellery, D.V.M., M.S.

ARTIFICIAL INSEMINATION and evaluation of semen quality are the 2 most common reasons for collection of stallion semen. In both of these cases it is advantageous to not contaminate the semen sample with the gel fraction of the ejaculate. The gel fraction hampers microscopic examination of the semen by impeding the motility of the spermatozoa and lowers the quality of the live-dead and morphology stains because the stain is prevented from coming into contact with the spermatozoa. The gel material may also occlude the syringe used for artificial insemination.

The artificial vagina has become an accepted means of collection of semen from the stallion. There are several equine artificial vaginas commercially available, but they are designed to collect the entire ejaculate, including the gel fraction. Using such collection devices, the gel fraction must be removed from the semen sample by filtering the sample through gauze after collection. This procedure is not only untidy, but also causes the loss of spermatozoa that become trapped in the gel material.

This report is a description of an equine artificial vagina modified in such a fashion that the gel fraction is retained in the artificial vagina so that it does not become part of the semen sample.

Description

In this laboratory a standard equine artificial vagina[a] is used as the basic piece of equipment for collection of semen samples from stallions. The material necessary for modification includes: (1) a wide-mouth, short-neck plastic funnel (3¼ in. wide, 4 in. high); (2) a piece of plastic tubing 20 cm. long[b]; and (3) 25 by 25 cm. squares of gauze[c] (Fig. 1).

The plastic tubing is attached to the small end of the funnel; 4 to 5 layers of gauze are placed over the large end of the funnel and held in place by adhesive tape around the outside of the funnel (Fig. 2). The funnel is inserted into the large end of the artificial vagina, tubing first, and pushed as far down into the cone of the artificial vagina as possible. At this point, the tubing will be protruding from the cone of the vagina approximately 5 cm. The tension of the cone of the artificial vagina is usually sufficient to hold the funnel in place, but a wide rubber band can be placed around the outside of the cone over the rim of the funnel if greater stability is desired.

The 250-ml. plastic collection bottle

Supported in part by the Victor Foundation, Chicago, Ill.

[a] Equine artificial vagina, horse size, Nasco, Fort Atkinson, Wis.

[b] Nalgon tubing, the Nalge Company, Inc., Rochester, N.Y.

[c] 28/24 mesh, Parke, Davis & Company, Detroit, Mich.

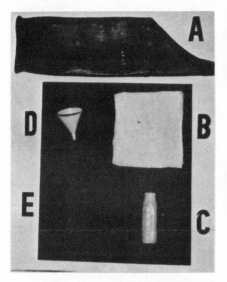

Fig. 1—Materials required to make the modified artificial vagina: artificial vagina (A); 3 to 4 layers of gauze, 25 by 25 cm. (B); plastic collection bottle (C); wide-mouth, short neck plastic funnel (D); plastic tubing (E).

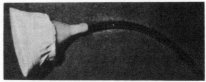

Fig. 2—Plastic funnel with gauze and plastic tubing attached. Apparatus is now ready to be placed in the artificial vagina.

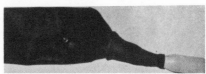

Fig. 3—Modified artificial vagina ready for collection of gel-free semen. Notice the wide rubber band holding the gauze-covered funnel in the neck of the artificial vagina.

that comes with the artificial vagina can next be attached to the vagina in the usual manner (Fig. 3). The plastic tubing will be protruding into the collection bottle. It is necessary to bore one or more holes in the upper part of the plastic bottle with a 16-gauge hypodermic needle to allow air to flow easily through the filter.

The modified artificial vagina is used in the usual manner.[2] When the stallion ejaculates, the presperm and sperm-rich fractions pass through the gauze, down the tube, and into the collection bottle. The gel fraction, which is ejaculated last,[1] is retained by the gauze and does not enter the sample.

Over 100 ejaculates have been collected from stallions in this laboratory, using this modified artificial vagina. In all cases, gel-free semen has been obtained.

References

1. Asdell, S. A.: Patterns of Mammalian Reproduction. 2nd ed. Cornell University Press, Ithaca, N.Y. (1964): 527.

2. Zemjanis, R.: Diagnostic and Therapeutic Techniques in Animal Reproduction. William and Wilkins Company, Baltimore, Md. (1962): 184.

ARTIFICIAL INSEMINATION IN THE EQUINE.
A COMPARISON OF NATURAL BREEDING AND ARTIFICIAL INSEMINATION OF MARES USING SEMEN FROM SIX STALLIONS

By JOHN P. HUGHES and ROBERT G. LOY

ARTIFICIAL insemination (AI) in the mare is a simple procedure but one which has seen limited use in the United States and certain parts of the world. In Russia[14] and China[8] it has been used extensively. Economic motivation to utilize AI in horse breeding in the United States is undoubtedly not so great as that related to cattle breeding because horse production here is primarily a hobby, or sports-related. Most horse breed organization rules either severely restrict or prohibit the exclusive use of artificial insemination.

It is not within the scope of this paper to present the pros and cons of AI in the horse industry. Because of the nature of the horse industry, not all of the advantages attributed to AI in other livestock programs apply. One obvious advantage in its use occurs when more than two mares need to be covered by a stallion within 1 day. An even more important reason for its use is the retention of valuable individuals in the breeding program that present serious impediments to its efficiency. These individuals include those mares with physical debilities which may virtually preclude natural matings, mares whose resistance to infection is markedly lowered,[11] or whose conformation is such that extensive suturing of the vulvar labia is necessary, mares that fail to show behavorial estrus, and mares whose cervices fail to dilate at estrus. In the latter case, "reinforcement" or "impregnation" with "tail-end samples" following natural cover is probably of little value. Stallions that harbor in their reproductive tracts organisms potentially pathogenic to mares that are susceptible to infections would be benefited by AI in that their semen might be pretreated with antibiotics included in semen extenders.[10]

This paper reports the use of two milk diluters for extending stallion semen and compares results of the use of extended semen with natural matings by the same stallions.

MATERIALS AND METHODS

The stallions used in this study were of the Thoroughbred and Quarterhorse breeds. The Thoroughbred stallions were from the experimental horse herd of the Animal Husbandry Department of the University of California at Davis and the Quarterhorse stallions were on breeding farms in the surrounding area.

The semen of the stallions was examined before the start of the breeding season and periodically during the breeding season. The reproductive classification of the stallion was based on its health, condition, libido and volume of ejaculate combined with microscopic examination of the spermatozoa for morphology and motility. Concentration of the semen sample and percentage of live spermatozoa were estimated under microscopic examination and only those samples judged to be abnormal were subjected to actual counts and vital staining. The semen of stallion no. 5 was classified only fair because of its low concentration and marginal percent of motile spermatozoa. Semen from the other five stallions was classified good.

All mares were subjected to regular teasing and rectal palpation of ovarian follicles to determine optimum time of breeding. A clinical evaluation of the reproductive health of the genitalia was made by examination of the cervix and vagina using a sterile glass speculum and by rectal palpation of the uterus. Cultures were taken from the cervices and uteri of mares in estrus when the clinical examination indicated the possibility of an infection. Only mares considered to be clinically normal and free of pathogens in the reproductive tract were bred naturally by the stallions. In a number of cases, mares with a history of genital infection or found to exhibit clinical evidence of infection on speculum examination were treated during the estrus at which they were artificially inseminated. Treatment was administered prior to insemination, both prior to insemination and following ovulation or only following ovulation.[11] A majority of mares artificially inseminated with semen from stallion no. 6 were in this class, although some were included among artificially inseminated mares for all stallions. Stallions and mares were brought to the breeding area and their external genitalia and surrounding skin were washed with Septisol,* rinsed, and wiped dry with a clean towel. Mares had their tails bandaged and were restrained by any of the conventional methods before being bred by the stallion or artificially inseminated. Collections of stallion semen were made using the artificial vagina as described in a previous article.[1] Semen was diluted immediately after collection.

The extenders used were skim milk and cream-gelatin. Skim milk diluter was prepared by warming skim milk in a double boiler to 95 C for 4 minutes. After the milk was cooled, 1,000 units of penicillin, 1 mg of dihydrostreptomycin and 200 units of Polymyxin B sulfate were added per ml of diluter. Cream-gelatin diluter was prepared by warming half-and-half cream in a double boiler to 95 C for 2 to 4 minutes. Any scum was removed and the hot half-and-half cream was added to

---

*Details on products and chemotherapeutic agents used in this study are given in the Appendix.

1.3 g. of Knox gelatin, which had been autoclaved with 10 ml of distilled water, to a volume of 100 ml.[17] When the mixture cooled, antibiotics were added as given for the skim milk diluter. Diluters were made up in advance and stored in a freezer until used.

Semen was diluted at the rate of 1 part semen to 1 part diluter or 1 part semen to 4 parts diluter. The diluter was warmed to 32 to 37 C before adding the semen and a volume of 50 ml was used to inseminate the mare. If used within 2 hours, diluted semen was not refrigerated; otherwise, it was cooled and stored at 0 to 5 C. Cooled semen was warmed to 32 to 37 C before it was deposited in the mare's uterus. Skim milk diluted semen was not kept past 24 hours. All inseminations after 24 hours were made using cream-gelatin diluted semen. Inseminations up to 24 hours were divided equally between skim milk and cream-gelatin diluted semen.

Artificial insemination was carried out by inserting a sterile glass speculum into the vagina, and a sterile Chambers catheter was then passed through the speculum and into the uterus by way of the cervix. A sterile 50-ml syringe filled with diluted semen was attached to the Chambers catheter and the mixture was deposited into the uterus. An alternate method was to direct the Chambers catheter through the cervix by inserting a hand encased in a sterile glove into the vagina.

RESULTS

A total of 218 mares was bred by artificial insemination and 199 by natural breeding. One hundred and forty-seven (67.4 percent) of the mares bred by artificial insemination conceived and 157 (78.9 percent) of the mares bred by natural breeding conceived. Twenty-seven of 37 (73.0 percent) mares inseminated with diluted semen stored at 0 to 5 C for 24 to 96 hours conceived (table I). Of these 37 mares, 10 of 14 conceived with semen inseminated after 24 hours' storage, 12 of 14 after 48 hours' storage, 3 of 6 after 72 hours' storage, and 2 of 3 after 96 hours' storage.

The following are the results obtained from individual stallions:

Stallion no. 1. Five of 10 (50.0 percent) mares artificially inseminated in 1960, 11 of 13 (84.6 percent) in 1961, and 23 of 29 (79.3 percent) in 1962 conceived. A total of 52 mares was artificially inseminated with semen from stallion no. 1 and 39 (75.0 percent) conceived (table II). It bred 26 mares

TABLE I

Status of mares artificially inseminated with diluted semen stored at 0 to 5 C for 24 to 96 hours

Hours stored	No. of mares	No. conceived	No. open
24	14	10	4
48	14	12	2
72	6	3	3
96	3	2	1
Totals	37	27	10

in 1960 and 20 (76.9) percent conceived, 34 in 1961 and 30 (88.2 percent) conceived, and 12 in 1962 and 9 (75.0 percent) conceived. A total of 72 mares was bred by natural breeding and 59 (81.9 percent) conceived (table III).

Stallion no. 2. One mare artificially inseminated in 1961, 11 of 13 (84.5 percent) in 1962, 17 of 21 (81.0 percent) in 1963, 8 of 10 (80.0 percent) in 1964, and 5 of 7 (71.4 percent) in 1965 conceived. A total of 52 mares was artificially inseminated with semen from stallion no. 2 and 42 (80.8 percent) conceived (table IV). It bred 4 mares in 1961 and 4 (100 percent) conceived, 16 in 1962 and 11 (68.7 percent) conceived, 16 in 1963 and 10 (62.5 percent) conceived, 5 in 1964 and 4 (80.0 percent) conceived, and 4 in 1965 and 4 (100 percent) conceived. A total of 45 mares was bred by natural breeding and 33 (73.3 percent) conceived (table V).

Stallion no. 3. Three of 3 mares artificially inseminated in 1963 and 3 of 6 mares (50.0 percent) in 1964 conceived. A total of 9 mares was artificially inseminated with semen from stallion no. 3 and 6 (66.6 percent) conceived (table VI). It bred 10 mares in 1963 and 6 (60.0 percent) conceived, and 11 in 1964 and 10 (90.9 percent) conceived. A total of 21 mares was bred by natural breeding and 16 (76.1 percent) conceived (table VII).

Stallion no. 4. Eight of 10 (80.0 percent) mares artificially inseminated in 1962, 5 of 10 (50.0 percent) in 1963, and 2 of 3 (66.6 percent) in 1964 conceived. A total of 23

TABLE II

Status of mares artifically inseminated with diluted semen from stallion no. 1

Year	Hr semen stored	No. of mares	No. conceived	No. open
1960	Under 2	10	5	5
1961	Under 2	10	9	1
	96	3	2	1
1962	Under 2	20	16	4
	24	7	6	1
	48	1	1	0
	96	1	0	1
	Totals	52	39	13

TABLE III

Status of mares bred to stallion no. 1

Year	No. of mares	No. conceived	No. open
1960	26	20	6
1961	34	30	4
1962	12	9	3
Totals	72	59	13

mares was artificially inseminated with semen from stallion no. 4 and 15 (65.2 percent) conceived (table VIII). It bred 5 mares in 1962 and 4 (80.0 percent) conceived, 25 in 1963 and 21 (84.0 percent) conceived, and 19 in 1964 and 16 (84.2 percent) conceived. A total of 49 mares was bred by natural breeding and 41 (83.7 percent) conceived (table IX).

Stallion no. 5. Nine of 16 (64.3 percent) mares artificially inseminated in 1964, 11 of 20 (55.0 percent) in 1965, and 13 of 16 (81.2 percent) in 1966 conceived. A total of 52 mares was artificially inseminated with semen from stallion no. 5 and 33 (63.5 percent) conceived (table X). It bred 1 mare in

1963 and 1 conceived, 7 in 1964 and 5 (71.4 percent) conceived, and 2 in 1965 and 1 (50.0 percent) conceived. A total of 10 mares was bred by natural breeding and 7 (70.0 percent) conceived (table XI).

Stallion no. 6. One mare artificially inseminated in 1964

TABLE IV

Status of mares artificially inseminated with diluted semen from stallion no. 2

Year	Hr semen stored	No. of mares	No. conceived	No. open
1961	Under 2	1	1	0
1962	Under 2	12	10	2
	48	1	1	0
1963	Under 2	17	14	3
	24	1	1	0
	72	3	2	1
1964	Under 2	3	2	1
	24	2	1	1
	48	5	5	0
1965	Under 2	6	4	2
	48	1	1	0
	Totals	52	42	10

TABLE V

Status of mares bred to stallion no. 2

Year	No. of mares	No. conceived	No. open
1961	4	4	0
1962	16	11	5
1963	16	10	6
1964	5	4	1
1965	4	4	0
Totals	45	33	12

TABLE VI

Status of mares artificially inseminated with diluted semen from stallion no. 3

Year	Hr semen stored	No. of mares	No. conceived	No. open
1963	Under 2	3	3	0
1964	Under 2	6	3	3
	Totals	9	6	3

failed to conceive. Eight of 18 mares (44.4 percent) artificially inseminated in 1965, and 4 of 11 (36.3 percent) in 1966 conceived. A total of 30 mares was artificially inseminated with

TABLE VII

Status of mares bred to stallion no. 3

Year	No. of mares	No. conceived	No. open
1963	10	6	4
1964	11	10	1
Totals	21	16	5

TABLE VIII

Status of mares artificially inseminated with diluted semen from stallion no. 4

Year	Hr semen stored	No. of mares	No. conceived	No. open
1962	Under 2	7	6	1
	48	2	2	0
	72	1	0	1
1963	Under 2	8	4	4
	24	1	0	1
	48	1	1	0
1964	Under 2	1	1	0
	48	2	1	1
	Totals	23	15	8

TABLE IX

Status of mares bred to stallion no. 4

Year	No. of mares	No. conceived	No. open
1962	5	4	1
1963	25	21	4
1964	19	16	3
Totals	49	41	8

semen from stallion no. 6 and 12 (40.0 percent) conceived (table XII). Only two mares were bred by natural breeding between 1964 and 1966, and one conceived.

DISCUSSION

A number of diluters have been suggested for prolonging

TABLE X

Status of mares artificially inseminated with diluted semen from stallion no. 5

Year	Hr semen stored	No. of mares	No. conceived	No. open
1964	Under 2	14	9	5
	24	1	0	1
	72	1	0	1
1965	Under 2	20	11	9
1966	Under 2	11	10	1
	24	2	1	1
	48	2	1	1
	72	1	1	0
	Totals	52	33	19

TABLE XI

Status of mares bred to stallion no. 5

Year	No. of mares	No. conceived	No. open
1963	1	1	0
1964	7	5	2
1965	2	1	1
Totals	10	7	3

TABLE XII

Status of mares artificially inseminated with diluted semen from stallion no. 6

Year	Hr semen stored	No. of mares	No. conceived	No. open
1964	Under 2	1	0	1
1965	Under 2	18	8	10
1966	Under 2	11	4	7
	Totals	30	12	18

the life of equine semen. One worker, using 5 percent glucose and 8 percent egg yolk as a diluter, listed an 85-percent conception rate for mares bred when the semen had been refrigerated 12 to 24 hours and a 72-percent conception rate when the semen had been refrigerated 48 hours.[5] Another diluter consisting of 1.4 parts glucose, 25 parts egg yolk, 100 parts sterilized whole cow milk, 50,000 IU penicillin and 0.5 g streptomycin was used at a dilution rate of 1 part semen and 2 parts diluter. After 48 hours the majority of the samples still showed 50 percent forward motility. Five mares which were inseminated conceived.[9] Still another suggestion is to dilute stallion semen at the rate of 1 part semen to 4 parts of diluter containing 5 g of powdered buttermilk and 5 g of glucose in 100 ml of double distilled water with the addition of 1 mg streptomycin and 400 IU of penicillin per ml.[4] The most extensive report indicated that milk powder diluters were superior to glucose or sucrose diluters.[8] A 10 percent solution was made from whole milk powder. The semen was diluted 1:5 or 1:10 and not less than 20 ml was used to inseminate each mare. A total of 100 million or more progressively motile spermatozoa was in each insemination. In 1959, approximately 600,000 mares were inseminated. The semen of each stallion was used to inseminate an average of 465 mares and the conception rate was listed as 61 percent. In 1960, they[4] used the semen from the two most popular stallions on 4,415 and 3,093 mares with conception rates of 76.9 and 68.1 percent, respectively.

A number of reports began to appear after 1956 on the successful storage of stallion semen by freezing.[12,13,17,20] One of the first published accounts of a mare conceiving after insemination with frozen semen was in 1957. Epididymal spermatozoa were used.[3] A Russian report in 1964 indicated a conception rate of 80 percent with semen stored at −79 C.[17] Commercial distribution of frozen semen was begun in California in 1968.* The company claimed a conception rate of 72 percent during field trials on 1,487 mares.

It is evident from the results obtained using artificial insemination in the equine that it can be a very successful method of getting mares of normal breeding health in foal,

*Horse Breeders Service, Inc., Petaluma, Calif.

and will probably maximize the chances of conceiving for infection-prone mares. In our studies, 147 of 218 (67.4 percent) mares bred by artificial insemination conceived and 157 of 199 (78.9 percent) mares bred by natural breeding conceived. It should be pointed out that the number of mares conceiving tends to be lower in the artificially inseminated group of mares because a number of mares that had been barren for several years were included in this group. Mares bred to three stallions (nos. 3, 5, and 6) on one farm illustrate this point. A total of 91 mares was artificially inseminated with semen from the three stallions and 51 (56.0 percent) conceived. Twenty-three of the 91 mares had been barren for several years. Eliminating the 23 infertile mares, we had 51 of 68 (75.0 percent) mares that became pregnant when artificially inseminated with semen from the three stallions. These stallions bred a total of 31 mares by natural breeding and 23 (74.2 percent) conceived.

It is very important that mares be inseminated at the proper time during estrus if a maximum number of pregnancies is to result. Estrus and ovulation data accumulated on a yearly basis for 7 years at the University of California indicate that the proportion of mares showing estrus of normal duration and accompanied by ovulation remains at a relatively constant 75 to 85 percent from April through October, but drops rapidly to a low 20 to 25 percent in January and February.[15] During January, February, and March, a high percentage of mares show great irregularity of all characteristics of the estrus cycle.

Mares in this study were teased daily or every other day. Rectal palpations of ovarian follicles were made during estrus to determine the optimum time to breed the mares. Artificial insemination or natural breeding was done within 48 hours of ovulation. In a few cases the mare was bred up to 12 hours past ovulation with good results.

In 1939 it was reported that 72.4 percent of 29 mares bred 6 to 14 hours after ovulation conceived, and it was concluded that there is no reason to fear a decrease in fertility in mares bred or inseminated shortly after ovulation.[18] In

1940, analysis of data from over 700 mares indicated that best results (85.6 to 87.6 percent) were obtained with insemination prior to ovulation. Insemination "during" ovulation resulted in a drop of 12 percent (63 mares) and 2 to 10 hours past ovulation resulted in a drop of 50 percent (44 mares) in the number that conceived.[19] In 1961, mares inseminated 48, 36 to 48, 24 to 36, 12 to 24, and 6 to 12 hours prior to ovulation had conception rates of 33.3, 66.2, 55.8, 78.1, and 100 percent, respectively. Insemination 6 hours after ovulation resulted in a conception rate of 85.7 percent.[8]

The use of artificial insemination in the horse in the United States is limited at the present time. It does not appear that the rules of any of the breed registries forbidding or limiting its application will be changed. Owners of grade mares make up the potential area of use, but the number of mares per owner is very small.

A serious problem with commercial artificial insemination in horses will be detection of estrus and follicle development in the mare to be inseminated, and unless this is done, poor conception rates will result.

SUMMARY

A comparison of natural breeding and artificial insemination of mares using semen from three Thoroughbred and three Quarterhorse stallions was made. One hundred and forty-seven of 218 (67.4 percent) mares bred by artificial insemination conceived and 157 of 199 (78.9 percent) mares bred by natural breeding conceived.

The semen extenders used were skim milk and cream-gelatin. Twenty-seven of 37 (73.0 percent) mares inseminated with diluted semen stored at 0 to 5 C for 24 to 96 hours conceived.

APPENDIX

Dihydrostreptomycin sulfate, E. R. Squibb & Sons, New York.

Knox gelatin, Knox Gelatin, Inc., Johnstown, N.Y.

Polymyxin B sulfate, The S. E. Massengill Co., Bristol, Tenn.

Potassium penicillin G, E. R. Squibb & Sons, New York.
Septisol: Antiseptic liquid soap (hexachlorophene 0.75
percent), Vestal Laboratories, St. Louis, Mo.

REFERENCES

1. Asbury, A. C., and J. P. Hughes. Use of the artificial vagina for equine semen collection. Jour. Amer. Vet. Med. Assoc., *144*, 879, 1964.
2. Arhipov, G. The dosage of semen in the artificial insemination of horses. Konevodstvo, *27*, 33, 1957. (Anim. Breed. Abs., *25*, 355, 1957.)
3. Barker, C. A. V., and J. C. C. Gandier. Pregnancy in a mare resulting from frozen epididymal spermatozoa. Canad. Jour. Compar. Med. and Vet. Sci., *21*, 47, 1957.
4. Berry, R. O., and P. J. Gazder. The viability of stallion spermatozoa as influenced by storage media and by antibiotics. Southwest Vet., *13*, 217, 1960.
5. Burko-Rogalevic, A. N. Storage of stallion semen for a long period. Konevodstvo, *5*, 27, 1949. (Anim. Breed. Abs., *18*, 41, 1950.)
6. Chao, T., and P.-H. Chang. An experimental report on the low temperature storage of stallion semen. Chin. Jour. Anim. Husb. and Vet. Sci., *1*, 5, 1962. (Anim. Breed. Abs., *32*, 445, 1964.)
7. Cheng, P.-L. The application of some investigations of reproductive physiology in horse breeding practice in China. Chin. Jour. Agr. Sci., *7*, 1, 1961. (Anim. Breed. Abs., *33*, 34, 1965.)
8. Cheng, P.-L. The present situation of artificial insemination of horses in China and some investigations on increasing conception rate of mares and breeding efficiency of stallions. Acta Vet. et Zootech. Sinica *5*, 29, 1962.
9. Ebertus, R. The dilution of stallion semen with whole cow milk. Monatsh f. VetMed., *17*, 618, 1962.
10. Hughes, J. P., A. C. Asbury, R. G. Loy, and H. E. Burd. The occurrence of *Pseudomonas* in the genital tract of stallions and its effect on fertility. Cornell Vet., *57*, 53, 1967.
11. Hughes, J. P., R. G. Loy, A. C. Asbury, and H. E. Burd. The occurrence of *Pseudomonas* in the reproductive tract of mares and its effect on fertility. Cornell Vet., *56*, 595, 1966.
12. Iljinskaja, T. The effect of various factors on stallion spermatozoa frozen to –70 C. Konevodstvo, *26*, 32, 1956. (Anim. Breed. Abs., *25*, 132, 1957.)
13. Krause, D., and D. Grove. Deep freezing of jackass and stallion semen in concentrated pellet form. Jour. Reprod. and Fert., *14*, 139, 1967.
14. Letard, E. L. Insemination artificielle, chez les animaux domestiques. Rec. de Méd. Vét., *111*, 683, 1935.
15. Loy, R. G. Unpublished data, 1970.
16. Rasbech, N. O. Suppleringskursus. I. Artificial insemination I. Hesteavlen, Royal Veterinary School, Denmark, 1959.
17. Rombe, S., V. Kotjagina, and N. Piler. An improved method for preserving semen at –79 C. Anim. Breed. Abs., *33*, 363, 1966.
18. Saltzman, A. A. Insemination of mares after ovulation. Sovetsk. Zootech., No. 4, 77, 1939. (Anim. Breed. Abs., *8*, 16, 1940.)
19. Zivotkov, H. I. The efficiency of mating and insemination of mares during or after ovulation. Sovetsk. Zootech., No. 1, 108, 1940. (Anim. Breed. Abs., *9*, 303, 1941.)
20. Zumarin, L. The storage of stallion semen by freezing. Konovodstvo, *29*, 24, 1959. (Anim. Breed. Abs., *27*, 282, 1960.)

Artificial Insemination in Sheep

FERTILIZATION AND SURVIVAL OF FERTILIZED EGGS IN THE EWE FOLLOWING SURGICAL INSEMINATION AT VARIOUS TIMES AFTER THE ONSET OF OESTRUS

By I. D. KILLEEN and N. W. MOORE

I. INTRODUCTION

Estimates of the fertilizable life of the ovine egg vary from 10 to 24 hr (Green and Winters 1935; Dauzier and Wintenberger 1952; Thibault 1967). The estimates have been obtained by mating at specific times after the onset of oestrus and the accuracy of the estimates must be dependent upon two assumptions. First, that ovulation occurs at a uniform time after the onset of oestrus, and second, that rate of transport of spermatozoa to the site of fertilization is uniformly rapid throughout oestrus. However, neither assumption appears to be strictly valid. Killeen and Moore (1970a) and Mattner and Braden (1969) have shown that the efficiency of transport of spermatozoa diminishes in late oestrus and individual variations in time elapsing between the onset of oestrus and ovulation have been well documented (Killeen 1969).

Capacitation of ram spermatozoa and the time taken for the process of capacitation to be completed could further affect estimates of the fertilizable life of the egg. However, Mattner (1963a) suggested that capacitation can be completed in the reproductive tract of the ewe in 1·5 hr. If capacitation is completed at a uniformly rapid rate throughout oestrus then there would be little effect upon estimates of fertilizable life.

The present study was designed to define the fertilizable life of the ovine egg and to investigate the effect of age of egg at the time of fertilization on its subsequent development.

II. Materials and Methods

A flock of 350 mature, cyclic, Merino ewes, 10 vasectomized rams, and 6 entire rams of proven fertility were used in two experiments (see following tabulations). The ewes were run with vasectomized rams and were inspected for oestrus at 3-hourly (experiment 1) or 6-hourly (experiment 2) intervals. The mid-point between successive inspections was taken as the mean time of onset of oestrus and subsequent time intervals were related to this estimated mean.

(a) Experiment 1

Ewes were inseminated either with pooled freshly ejaculated semen which had been collected by artificial vagina from at least three rams, or similar semen after it had been incubated for 6 hr in ligated fallopian tubes of oestrous ewes. Animals used for incubation had been first detected in oestrus no more than 12 hr previous to incubation. A ligature was placed around the tube adjacent to the utero-tubal junction and $0 \cdot 2$–$0 \cdot 3$ ml fresh semen was injected through the fimbria, and another ligature was secured around the tube adjacent to the fimbria. Semen was recovered by removing the fimbria ligature, a polythene cannula was inserted into the tube, and the semen was exhausted through the cannula by flushing with 1 ml normal saline injected into the tube near the utero-tubal junction. Only those samples which contained progressively motile spermatozoa were used for insemination.

Inseminations were carried out under general anaesthesia (Nembutal) and semen was deposited into the ampulla of the tubes or tip of the uterine horns corresponding to ovaries containing a recent ovulation or finite follicle. Irrespective of type of semen used similar volumes were placed in each tube ($0 \cdot 01$ ml) or uterine horn ($0 \cdot 05$ ml). All ewes were laparotomized 27 hr after the time of insemination and the fallopian tubes and portion of the uterine horns were flushed with cold normal saline. Eggs recovered from the flushings were examined as unstained preparations.

A summary of the design of experiment 1 is set out in the following tabulation:

(1) Time of insemination (hr after onset of oestrus $\pm 1 \cdot 5$ hr)—30 v. 36 v. 42 v. 48 v. 54;

(2) Treatment of semen—nil v. incubated;

(3) Site of insemination—uterus v. fallopian tube.

Factorial: $5 \times 2 \times 2$: $n = 4$ ewes; total ewes $= 80$.

(b) Experiment 2

Inseminations using pooled freshly ejaculated semen were made into the cervix ($0 \cdot 20$ ml) or uterine horns ($0 \cdot 05$ ml) in ewes 12–48 hr after they were first detected in oestrus. Uterine inseminations were carried out as in experiment 1, whilst standard non-surgical techniques were used for cervical inseminations.

Following insemination the ewes were either allowed to go to term or they were laparotomized for egg recovery at 30 hr after insemination (ewes inseminated at 24, 36, and 48 hr after the onset of oestrus) or at 42 hr after insemination (ewes inseminated at 12 hr). These times were adopted to ensure that the majority of fertilized ova would have cleaved at least once when recovered. The eggs were examined as unstained preparations and again after staining with 1% orcein. The design of experiment 2 may be summarized as follows:

(1) Time of insemination (hr after onset of oestrus ± 3 hr)—12 v. 24 v. 36 v. 48;

(2) Site of insemination—cervix v. uterus;

(3) Fate of ewes—egg recovery v. lambing.

Factorial: $4 \times 2 \times 2$; $n = 12$ ewes; total ewes $= 192$.

73

(c) *General*

In both experiments ewes from which no eggs were recovered were replaced by animals in which egg recovery was successful. In experiment 1 in which eggs were examined as unstained preparations, the only available criterion of fertilization was that of apparently normal cleavage, whereas in experiment 2 examination of eggs after staining with orcein enabled a critical assessment to be made of the cytological state of cleaved and uncleaved eggs.

(d) *Statistical Procedures*

Where group sizes were equal, standard analyses of variance were applied to the raw or appropriately transformed data. With unequal sized groups, analyses of χ^2 were applied to the raw data. The analyses were carried out using a computer program (CHIPARTIN; control data 3600, Canberra) which enabled the partitioning for main effects and interactions into comparisons based on individual degrees of freedom, using orthogonal polynomial coefficients weighted according to the group size for each factor level (Claringbold 1961).

III. Results

(a) *Experiment 1*

A total of 123 ewes were inseminated and all but two had ovulated at the time of insemination. The two ewes were inseminated at 30 hr and when laparotomized for

TABLE 1

EXPERIMENT 1: NUMBER OF EWES WHICH YIELDED EGGS FOLLOWING UTERINE AND TUBAL INSEMINATION

Main effects. There were no significant interactions

Main Effect	No. of Ewes Inseminated	No. which Yielded Eggs	No. which Yielded Cleaved Eggs*	No. which Yielded Uncleaved Eggs — With Spermatozoa Attached	No. which Yielded Uncleaved Eggs — Without Spermatozoa Attached	Total No. of Eggs Recovered
1. Time of insemination (hr)†						
30	20	16	9 (2)	3	4	18
36	24	16‡	10	0	5	16
42	24	15	10	1	4	15
48	24	16	7	8	1	16
54	31	16	3	7	6	16
P (linear)		n.s.	$< 0\cdot05$	$< 0\cdot01$	n.s.	
P (remainder)		n.s.	n.s.	n.s.	n.s.	
2. Treatment of semen						
Nil	65	40‡	24 (1)	9	6	41
Incubated	58	39	15 (1)	10	14	40
P		n.s.	$< 0\cdot05$	n.s.	$< 0\cdot05$	
3. Site of insemination						
Uterus	51	39‡	20 (1)	8	10	40
Tubes	72	40	19 (1)	11	10	41
P		$< 0\cdot05$	n.s.	n.s.	n.s.	
Total	123	79†	39 (2)	19	20	81

* Number of ewes which yielded two eggs shown in parenthesis.

† Hours after onset of oestrus.

‡ One fractured egg recovered from one ewe—no cleavage data available.

egg recovery 27 hr later, both had ovulated. Eggs were recovered from 79 of the 123 ewes and there was an effect of site of insemination on egg recovery (Table 1). Six ewes had two ovulations, the remainder were monovular. Two eggs were recovered from two of the six ewes and all four eggs had cleaved.

The low incidence of cleaved eggs in ewes inseminated at 48 and 54 hr was associated with an increase in the number of uncleaved eggs with spermatazoa attached to their zonae pellucidae. Incubation of semen decreased the number of ewes with cleaved eggs and increased the incidence of uncleaved eggs without spermatozoa attached to their zonae pellucidae.

Of the 41 cleaved eggs that were recovered 31 were of two cells and the remainder were of three or four cells, but there was no effect of any treatment on cell stage. Three eggs showed unequal cleavage. They had one or more small cells associated with apparently normal-sized blastomeres (Fig. 1).

(b) *Experiment 2*

(i) *Egg Recovery*

Information on the time of ovulation was provided by the four groups of ewes which were surgically inseminated 12, 24, 36, and 48 hr after the onset of oestrus. Ovulation was first recorded at 24 hr and by 36 hr all ewes had ovulated, as shown in the following tabulation:

Time of insemination (hr):	12	24	36	48
No. of ewes inseminated:	26	29	26	31
No. of ewes which ovulated:	0	22	26	31

At 24 hr all ewes that had not yet ovulated showed well-defined follicles and ovulation appeared to be imminent. In order to obtain 96 successful egg recoveries 118 ewes had

TABLE 2

EXPERIMENT 2: NUMBER OF EWES WHICH YIELDED EGGS FOLLOWING CERVICAL AND UTERINE INSEMINATION

Main effects

Main Effect	No. of Ewes Insemin- ated	No. which Yielded Eggs	No. which Yielded Fertilized Eggs		Total No. of Eggs Recovered
			Normal*	Abnormal	
Time of insemination (hr)†					
12	27	24	24 (2)	0	26
24	31	24	20 (1)	0	25
36	27	24	9	4	27
48	33	24	4 (1)	6	26
P (linear)		n.s.	< 0·001	< 0·05	
P (remainder)		n.s.	n.s.	n.s.	
Site of insemination					
Cervix	54	48	20 (1)	1	51
Uterus	64	48	37 (3)	9	53
P		n.s.	< 0·001	< 0·05	
Total	118	96	57 (4)	10	104

* No. of ewes which yielded two fertilized eggs are shown in parenthesis.
† Hours after onset of oestrus.

to be inseminated (Table 2). Two eggs were recovered from 8 of 10 ewes which shed two eggs. The remaining ewes were monovular. Of the 104 eggs that were recovered,

75

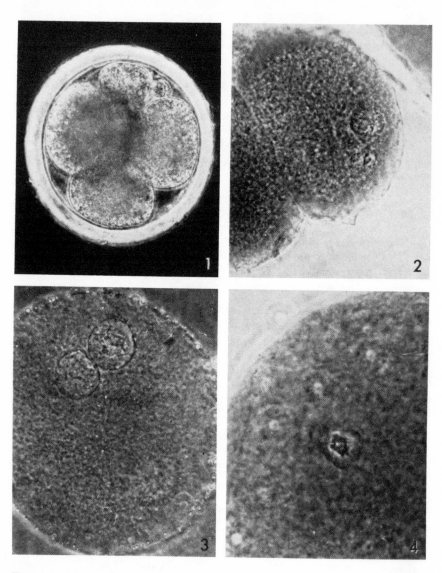

Fig. 1.—An atypical (type 1) four-cell egg with three small "cells" associated with four apparently normal blastomeres. Fresh preparation. × 280.

Fig. 2.—An abnormal (type 2) two-cell egg showing a large nucleus and several subnuclei in one blastomere. Orcein-stained. × 280.

Fig. 3.—An abnormal (type 3) one-cell egg which contained three pronuclei (two only in focal plane). Orcein-stained. × 280.

Fig. 4.—An aged, unfertilized egg recovered 66 hr after the onset of oestrus. Note compact appearance of the female nucleus. Orcein-stained. × 600.

33 showed no evidence of penetration or activation by spermatozoa. The chromatin of unfertilized eggs was characteristically compact (Fig. 4) and, except for one egg recovered following uterine insemination at 48 hr, no spermatozoa were found attached to the zonae pellucidae of unfertilized eggs. The remaining 71 eggs were fertilized; 62 had cleaved at least once while nine were of one cell and contained at least two well-formed pronuclei. Where two eggs were recovered from individual ewes both were either fertilized or unfertilized.

Three types of eggs of unusual appearance were recorded:

Type 1: Eggs with anucleate particles generally smaller than normal blastomeres (Fig. 1)—15 eggs.

Type 2: Individual blastomeres with more than one nucleus (Fig. 2)—7 eggs.

Type 3: Eggs of one cell with more than two pronuclei (Fig. 3)—3 eggs.

The occurrence of all three types of eggs was more common following uterine insemination. Of the 25 eggs involved, all but two were recovered after uterine insemination. Type 1 eggs were "atypical" rather than abnormal and for the purposes of statistical analyses they have been considered to be normal fertilized eggs. Types 2 and 3 showed gross nuclear aberrations and have been considered to be abnormal fertilized eggs.

There were marked effects of site of insemination and of time of insemination on the proportion of ewes which yielded normal fertilized eggs (Table 2) and a large portion of these effects was due to the complete absence of normal fertilized eggs in ewes cervically inseminated at 36 and 48 hr after the onset of oestrus (Table 3).

TABLE 3

EXPERIMENT 2: NUMBER OF EWES WITH NORMAL FERTILIZED EGGS OR LAMBS FOLLOWING EITHER CERVICAL OR UTERINE INSEMINATION

$n = 12$

Time of Insemination (hr)*	Cervical Insemination			Uterine Insemination			Totals	
	No. with Fertilized Eggs	No. with Lambs	Total	No. with Fertilized Eggs	No. with Lambs	Total	With Fertilized Eggs	With Lambs
12	12	8	20	12	4	16	24	12
24	8	3	11	12	1	13	20	4
36	0	0	0	9	1	10	9	1
48	0	0	0	4	0	4	4	0
Total	20	11	31	37	6	43	57	17

Significant main effects	Significant interactions
Time of insemination (linear): $P < 0.001$	Site of insemination $\times$ fate of ewes: $P < 0.001$
Site of insemination (cervix v. uterus): $P < 0.05$	Time of insemination $\times$ fate: $P < 0.05$
Fate of ewes (fertile v. lambed): $P < 0.001$	Time $\times$ site: $P < 0.05$

* Hours after onset of oestrus.

(ii) *Lambing Performance*

Only 17 of 96 ewes allowed to go to term lambed and when fertilization and lambing data were compared major discrepancies were observed (Table 3). The

77

difference between fertilization and lambing performance was most marked following uterine insemination. Of 48 ewes cervically inseminated 20 gave fertilized eggs and 11 of 48 lambed, whereas following uterine insemination 37 ewes had fertilized eggs but only 6 lambed. The effect of time of insemination on fertilization was somewhat different from its effect on lambing performance and the effect of time of insemination was further modified by site of insemination. There was complete failure of normal fertilization and lambing in ewes cervically inseminated at 36 and 48 hr after the onset of oestrus, whereas with uterine insemination at 36 and 48 hr some ewes had normal fertilized eggs (nine and four), but only one ewe lambed.

IV. DISCUSSION

Both experiments provided information on the time of ovulation and on the fertilizable life of the ovine egg. In experiment 2 the majority of ewes had ovulated by 24 hr after the onset of oestrus and by 30 hr in experiment 1 ovulation was almost complete. Assuming that the majority of ewes ovulated about 24 hr after the onset of oestrus then experiment 1 showed that eggs remained highly fertile for 12–18 hr. No decrease in the number of ewes with cleaved eggs occurred until 48 hr had elapsed between the onset of oestrus and insemination. It is possible that the fertilization process in the older eggs was somewhat retarded and a number of uncleaved eggs recovered after insemination at 48 and 54 hr may have been fertilized. However, in experiment 2 in which eggs of a similar age were subjected to more critical examination only 9 of 42 uncleaved eggs had been fertilized.

Experiment 1 did not provide any positive evidence on the need for capacitation of ram spermatozoa. If capacitation is necessary and can be achieved in 1·5 hr (Mattner 1963a) then it is unlikely that the cell stage of fertilized eggs is sufficiently critical to detect differences in the rapidity of penetration and activation of eggs by incubated and non-incubated spermatozoa. Tubal incubation, as in the rabbit, may not efficiently capacitate spermatozoa (Adams and Chang 1962). The fallopian tubes do not provide a favourable environment for the survival of ram spermatozoa (Quinlan, Maré, and Roux 1933; Mattner 1963b). The lowered incidence of cleaved eggs and the relatively high incidence of cleaved eggs without spermatozoa attached to their zonae pellucidae which were associated with the use of incubated spermatozoa would indicate a loss of viability during incubation in the tubes.

Surgical insemination either into the fallopian tubes or the uterus as late as 54 hr after the onset of oestrus gave some fertilization, but there was almost complete failure of fertilization with cervical insemination carried out later than 24 hr after the onset of oestrus. Similarly, no ewe inseminated cervically at 36 and 48 hr subsequently lambed. It seems likely as suggested by Mattner and Braden (1969) and shown by Killeen and Moore (1970a) that faulty transport of spermatozoa from the cervix to the tubes in late oestrus was responsible for failure of fertilization in late cervically inseminated ewes.

Surgical insemination resulted in a number of eggs of unusual appearance. In experiment 1 the only "unusual" eggs that could be detected were those which had small particles associated with normal-sized blastomeres. The staining procedures used in experiment 2 showed that these particles were devoid of nuclei. Further and probably more serious nuclear abnormalities were detected in experiment 2 (types 2 and 3). Type 2 and type 3 eggs were almost invariably associated with late uterine insemination whilst those of type 1 were distributed at random throughout the various times of insemination. Although the present experiments provide no direct evidence on the viability of these eggs, it has been shown that eggs of type 1 are capable of full development (Hancock and Hovell 1961; and Killeen and Moore 1970b) and should therefore be classed as "atypical" rather than abnormal. The severe nuclear aberrations of type 2 and type 3 eggs probably preclude full development and as in other species (see Hunter 1967) they resulted from the exposure of "aged" eggs to spermatozoa. Faulty transport of spermatozoa in ewes inseminated late in oestrus would not allow fertilization of aged eggs. Thus under normal conditions of natural service and artificial insemination it is doubtful if these types of severe nuclear abnormalities play any significant part in reproductive wastage.

Loss of abnormal eggs of types 2 and 3 could be responsible for some, but certainly not all, of the difference between fertilization and lambing performance following uterine insemination. Similar discrepancies have been observed by Salamon and Lightfoot (1967) and it now appears that loss of fertilized eggs following uterine (or tubal) insemination is due to excessively rapid transport of eggs within the reproductive tract (Killeen and Moore 1970b).

V. Acknowledgments

Grateful acknowledgment for technical assistance is made to Dr. T. D. Quinlivan, Mr. A. D. Barnes, Mr. R. J. Maddy, and Mrs. Margaret Jeffrey.

Financial support was provided by the Australian Research Grants Committee and the Australian Wool Board. One of us (I.D.K.) was the recipient of a Wool Board Post-Graduate Fellowship.

VI. References

ADAMS, C. E., and CHANG, M. C. (1962).—Capacitation of rabbit spermatozoa in the Fallopian tube and in the uterus. *J. exp. Zool.* **151**, 159.

CLARINGBOLD, P. J. (1961).—The use of orthogonal polynomials in the partition of chi-square. *Aust. J. Statist.* **3**, 48.

DAUZIER, L., and WINTENBERGER, S. (1952).—Recherches sur la fécondation chez les mammifères. Durée du pouvoir fécondant des spermatozoïdes de bélier dans le tractus génital de la brebis et durée de la periode de fécondité de l'oeuf après l'ovulation. *C.r. Séanc. Soc. Biol.* **146**, 660.

GREEN, W. W., and WINTERS, L. M. (1935).—Studies on the physiology of reproduction in the sheep. III. The time of ovulation and rate of sperm travel. *Anat. Rec.* **61**, 457.

HANCOCK, J. L., and HOVELL, G. J. R. (1961).—Transfer of sheep ova. *J. Reprod. Fert.* **2**, 520.

HUNTER, R. H. F. (1967).—The effects of delayed insemination on fertilization and early cleavage in the pig. *J. Reprod. Fert.* **13**, 133.

KILLEEN, I. (1969).—Studies in fertilization and early development of the ovine ovum. Ph. D. Thesis, University of Sydney.

KILLEEN, I. D., and MOORE, N. W. (1970a).—Transport of spermatozoa, and fertilization in the ewe following cervical and uterine insemination early and late in oestrus. *Aust. J. biol. Sci.* **23**, 1271.

KILLEEN, I. D., and MOORE, N. W. (1970b).—The morphological appearance and development of sheep ova fertilized by surgical insemination. *J. Reprod. Fert.* (In press.)

MATTNER, P. E. (1963a).—Capacitation of ram spermatozoa and penetration of the ovine egg. *Nature, Lond.* **199**, 772.

MATTNER, P. E. (1963b).—Spermatozoa in the genital tract of the ewe. III. The role of spermatozoan motility and of uterine contractions in transport of spermatozoa. *Aust. J. biol. Sci.* **16**, 877.

MATTNER, P. E., and BRADEN, A. W. H. (1969).—Effect of time of insemination on the distribution of spermatozoa in the genital tract in ewes. *Aust. J. biol. Sci.* **22**, 1283.

QUINLAN, J., MARÉ, G. S., and ROUX, L. L. (1933).—A study of the duration of motility of spermatozoa in the different divisions of the reproductive tract of the Merino ewe. *Onderstepoort J. vet. Sci. Anim. Ind.* **1**, 135.

SALAMON, S., and LIGHTFOOT, R. J. (1967).—Fertilization and embryonic loss in sheep after insemination with deep frozen semen. *Nature, Lond.* **216**, 194.

THIBAULT, C. (1967).—Analyse comparée de la fécondation et de ses anomalies chez la brebis, la vache et la lapine. *Annls Biol. anim. Biochim. Biophys.* **7**, 5.

THE MORPHOLOGICAL APPEARANCE AND DEVELOPMENT OF SHEEP OVA FERTILIZED BY SURGICAL INSEMINATION

I. D. KILLEEN AND N. W. MOORE

INTRODUCTION

Surgical insemination of the ewe, involving the direct injection of semen into either the Fallopian tubes or the uterine horns, has been shown to give high rates of fertilization but subsequent lambing performances have been poor (Salamon & Lightfoot, 1967; Mattner, Entwistle & Martin, 1969; Killeen,

1969). Salamon & Lightfoot (1967) and Mattner *et al.* (1969) suggested that the differences between fertilization and lambing were due to excessive embryonic loss. However, their studies provided no direct evidence on the fate of eggs fertilized by surgical insemination.

Either or both of two explanations may account for the large discrepancy between fertilization and lambing performances, namely, the direct effects of surgical insemination on the egg or on the genital tract.

The first explanation gains some support from the work of Killeen (1969), who found that a number of eggs fertilized by surgical insemination contained small anucleate particles. The incidence of these so-called 'abnormal' eggs could account for some, but not all, of the difference between fertilization and lambing performance. However, the study provided no direct evidence on the viability of the 'abnormal' eggs. Surgical insemination places all the components of semen within close proximity of recently ovulated eggs and it is possible that components which are normally lost or diluted during passage from the vagina to the tubes are present in sufficient concentration to have a deleterious effect upon the viability of fertilized eggs. In the rabbit, there is suggestive evidence that high concentrations of seminal plasma can affect the development of fertilized eggs (Chang, 1950; Hadek, 1959). Freshly ejaculated semen probably contains a number of spermatozoa, which by nature of their age and other characteristics may be classed as only partially competent. Such spermatozoa may well lose their viability during passage through the tract but, with surgical insemination, they could actively compete with 'fully competent' spermatozoa. Eggs fertilized by partially competent spermatozoa, however, may not possess the capacity for full development.

The second explanation depends upon the assumption that surgery and the consequent manipulation of the tract result in failure of eggs to enter the Fallopian tubes or in rapid transport of fertilized eggs to the uterus, a site known to provide an environment unfavourable for 'underdeveloped' eggs (Averill & Rowson, 1958; Moore & Shelton, 1964).

MATERIALS AND METHODS

Experimental animals and design

A flock of 500 mature cyclic Merino ewes, sixteen vasectomized rams and six entire rams of proven fertility were used in two experiments designed to study the morphological appearance and the subsequent development of eggs fertilized by uterine insemination. The ewes were run with the vasectomized rams and they were inspected for oestrus twice daily at 06.00 and 18.00 hours.

The design of the experiments is shown in Table 1. Fertilized eggs were collected from donor ewes which had been previously treated with 1000 to 1200 i.u. pregnant mare's serum gonadotrophin on the 12th to 14th day of the oestrous cycle and the eggs were either examined after staining with 1 % orcein, or they were transferred to recipient ewes. In Exp. 1, embryos were recovered on the 16th day after oestrus, while in Exp. 2, recipients were allowed to go to term.

Apart from those animals in Exp. 2 which were naturally mated, donors were surgically inseminated into the tip of the uterine horns with (a) 'fresh semen', (b) 'washed semen' or (c) 'uterine semen'.

'Washed semen' was prepared in Exp. 1 by repeated washing and centrifuging with calcium-free Krebs–Ringer phosphate solution (0·01 M-Na_2HPO_4, 0·005 M-KCl, 0·001 M-KH_2PO_4, 0·001 M-$MgSO_4$, 0·132 M-NaCl) or with normal saline in Exp. 2. To 0·5 ml of fresh semen collected by artificial vagina was added 9·5 ml diluent, the sample was centrifuged at 1500 rev/min for 10 min and 9 ml of the supernatant was then removed and replaced with fresh diluent. The sedimented spermatozoa were resuspended by shaking and again centrifuged. This procedure was repeated a further four times. The sedimented 'semen' obtained after the final centrifugation was used for insemination.

TABLE 1

DESIGN OF THE EXPERIMENTS

Treatment of semen before insemination	No. of fertilized eggs	
	Stained*	Transferred to recipient ewes
Experiment 1		
1. 'Fresh semen'—freshly ejaculated	20	19
2. 'Washed semen'—washed with calcium-free Krebs–Ringer solution	21	20
3. 'Uterine semen'—recovered from naturally mated ewes	18	18
Experiment 2		
1. 'Fresh semen'—freshly ejaculated	14	29
2. 'Washed semen'—washed with normal saline	11	28
3. 'Uterine semen'—recovered from naturally mated ewes	19	40
4. Nil—donors naturally mated	21	35
Total	124	189

* Fate of recipients: Exp. 1—embryos recovered; Exp. 2—lambed.

'Uterine semen' was obtained by flushing the Fallopian tubes and uterine horns of the naturally mated ewes with 10 ml of calcium-free Krebs–Ringer phosphate solution (Exp. 1) or normal saline (Exp. 2). The flushings were centrifuged at 1500 rev/min for 10 min and the supernatant was removed to leave 0·2 to 0·4 ml of diluent and sediment. The sediment was resuspended in the remaining diluent and a small sample was taken for examination. A number of samples which contained few, or no, progressively motile spermatozoa were discarded.

Ewes were inseminated under local Xylocaine anaesthesia, 12 to 27 hr after they were first observed in oestrus. No attempt was made to control the number of spermatozoa inseminated. Each ewe received 0·02 to 0·04 ml semen irrespective of its treatment and inseminations were made into both uterine horns with the volume of inseminate approximately equally divided between each horn.

Recovery of eggs

Eggs were recovered by flushing the Fallopian tubes and portions of the uterine horns of donor ewes with sterile sheep serum 60 hr after they were first detected in oestrus. This interval was adopted to ensure that the majority of fertilized eggs had cleaved at least once by the time they were recovered. Cleavage was taken as the criterion of fertilization and fertilized eggs collected from individual donors were approximately equally divided between those destined for cytological examination and those destined for transfer. An attempt was made to attain uniform numbers of eggs within groups. However, variations in numbers of eggs recovered, or in numbers of eggs fertilized, made impractical the achievement of uniform group size.

Examination of eggs

Cleaved eggs destined for cytological study were examined as unstained preparations and then were re-examined after staining with 1 % orcein. They were classed as normal or abnormal:

Normal   All cells of approximately equal size, with one nucleus in each cell.

Abnormal   Type 1. Anucleate particles present.
            Type 2. Multinucleate cells present.

All one-cell eggs recovered from donor ewes were examined for evidence of fertilization.

Transfer of eggs

Transfers were made to the Fallopian tubes of recipient ewes which had been first observed in oestrus within ± 12 hr of their respective donors, and each recipient received one egg. Recoveries and transfers were carried out under general anaesthesia with Nembutal.

Recovery of embryos

Embryos were recovered from recipients on the 16th day after the transfer oestrus (i.e. 13 to 14 days after transfer) by flushing the uteri *in vivo* with 10 ml normal saline. The flushings were collected through a 5-mm bore glass cannula inserted into the tip of one uterine horn. Embryos and their associated membranes were examined under a dissecting microscope ($\times 20$ magnification).

Lambing

During lambing, the recipients were inspected at least once daily and newly born lambs were identified.

TABLE 2

EGGS RECOVERED AND EGGS FERTILIZED FOLLOWING INSEMINATION OF DONOR EWES WITH TREATED SEMEN

Treatment of semen	Method of insemination	Experiment 1					Experiment 2				
		No. of ewes		No. of eggs shed	% Recovered	% Fertilized	No. of ewes		No. of eggs shed	% Recovered	% Fertilized
		Inseminated	Yielded eggs				Inseminated	Yielded eggs			
'Fresh'	Uterine	18	15	70	61	98	12	12	80	68	96
'Washed'	Uterine	18	18	67	75	94	14	12	92	54	88
'Uterine'	Uterine	36	36	113	73	49	28	26	152	68	61
Nil	Naturally mated	—	—	—	—	—	12	12	78	86	93
Total		72	69	250	70	74	66	62	402	68	81

Proportion of eggs shed that were recovered—Exp. 1: $\chi^2_3 = 3.51$; NS. Exp. 2: $\chi^2_3 = 19.41$; $P < 0.001$.
Proportion of recovered eggs that were fertilized—Exp. 1: $\chi^2_3 = 49.68$; $P < 0.001$. Exp. 2: $\chi^2_3 = 41.34$; $P < 0.001$.

TABLE 3

NORMAL AND ABNORMAL CLEAVED EGGS RECOVERED FOLLOWING INSEMINATION OF DONOR EWES WITH TREATED SEMEN

Treatment of semen	Method of insemination	Experiment 1					Experiment 2				
		No. of normal eggs	No. of abnormal eggs		% total abnormal eggs	Total no. of eggs	No. of normal eggs	No. of abnormal eggs		% total abnormal eggs	Total no. of eggs
			Type 1	Type 2				Type 1	Type 2		
'Fresh'	Uterine	9	11	0	55	20	7	6	1	50	14
'Washed'	Uterine	12	9	0	43	21	10	1	0	9	11
'Uterine'	Uterine	5	12	1	72	18	8	11	0	58	19
Nil	Naturally mated	—	—	—	—	—	6	15	0	71	21
Total		26	32	1	56	59	31	33	1	52	65

Proportion of cleaved eggs that were classed as abnormal (Type 1+Type 2)—Exp. 1: $\chi^2_3 = 3.40$; NS. Exp. 2: $\chi^2_3 = 11.72$; $P < 0.01$.

RESULTS

In the two experiments, 449 eggs were recovered from 131 of 138 donor ewes (Table 2). In Exp. 1, there was no effect of any treatment on the proportion of eggs that were recovered while, in Exp. 2, there was an effect of treatment ($P<0\cdot001$) due to the high rate of recovery (86%) from naturally mated donors. In both experiments, there was a marked reduction in the proportion of eggs that were fertilized following insemination with 'uterine semen'.

Ninety-nine uncleaved eggs were recovered, of which eighty-two were from ewes inseminated with 'uterine semen'. Only eight had spermatozoa attached to their zonae, of which five showed definite evidence of penetration by spermatozoa. None of the remaining eggs showed any evidence of having been fertilized.

The cell stage of the 350 fertilized cleaved eggs ranged from two to eight cells with the majority (301) of four to eight cells. There was no effect of any treatment on the distribution of cell stage.

TABLE 4

RECIPIENTS WHICH HAD EMBRYOS OR LAMBS FOLLOWING THE TRANSFER OF CLEAVED EGGS COLLECTED FROM EWES INSEMINATED WITH TREATED SEMEN

Treatment of semen	Method of insemination	Recipients			
		Experiment 1		Experiment 2	
		Total no.	% with an embryo	Total no.	% which lambed
'Fresh'	Uterine	19	63	29	59
'Washed'	Uterine	20	45	28	43
'Uterine'	Uterine	18	33	40	53
Nil	Naturally mated	—	—	35	51
Total		57	47	132	52

Proportion of recipients in which eggs survived—Exp. 1: $\chi^2_2 = 3\cdot27$; NS. Exp. 2: $\chi^2_3 = 1\cdot44$; NS.

Examination of eggs

Twenty-four cleaved eggs were lost or fractured before examination was completed and have been excluded from the experiment. In all, sixty-seven of the 124 cleaved eggs available for morphological study were classed as 'abnormal' (Table 3). Sixty-five contained one or more anucleate particles (Type 1—Pl. 1, Figs. 1 to 3) and the remaining two had one multinucleate cell.

Frequently, Type 1 eggs contained more than one anucleate particle, but these were invariably associated with normal nucleated blastomeres. The size of particles varied from that of a polar body to that of a normal blastomere. Type 1 'abnormal' eggs invariably showed nothing more unusual than one or more anucleate particles.

In Exp. 1, 'abnormal' eggs were equally distributed between the various

86

PLATE 1

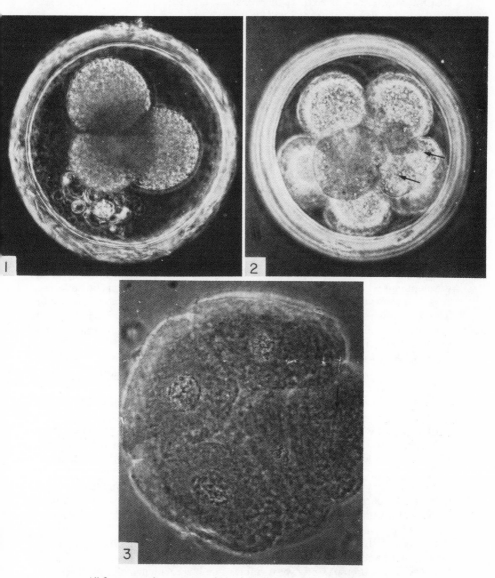

All figures are phase contrast photomicrographs of abnormal (Type 1) eggs.

FIG. 1. A four-cell egg which contained numerous small anucleate particles. Fresh preparation, × 280.

FIG. 2. A seven-cell egg which contained five anucleate particles. Two of the particles (arrowed) can be distinguished in the photograph. Fresh preparation, × 280.

FIG. 3. A four-cell egg which contained an anucleate particle (arrowed). Orcein stained preparation, × 140.

treatments, whereas, in Exp. 2, there was an effect of treatment due to a low incidence in ewes inseminated with 'washed semen'.

Development following transfer

In Exp. 1, twenty-seven of fifty-seven ewes had embryos and, in Exp. 2, sixty-eight of 132 recipients lambed (Table 4). None of the embryos or lambs showed any obvious abnormalities and there was no effect of any treatment on the proportion of eggs which survived to become embryos or lambs.

DISCUSSION

Apart from ewes inseminated with 'uterine semen', very high rates of fertilization were achieved by uterine insemination. It is apparent that low lambing performances reported following uterine insemination (Salamon & Lightfoot, 1967; Mattner et al., 1969; Killeen, 1969) are not due to failure of fertilization. The low fertilization rates recorded in both experiments following insemination with 'uterine semen' were probably due to the poor quality of the semen. A number of samples used, particularly in Exp. 1, contained few progressively motile spermatozoa.

Eggs fertilized by uterine insemination were viable and capable of normal development when transferred to recipients. Although the survival of transferred eggs was somewhat lower than could be expected (Moore & Rowson, 1960; Moore & Shelton, 1964), the proportion that did develop to become normal embryos or lambs was not affected by the method of insemination, or by treatment of semen before surgical insemination.

More than half of the eggs examined were classed as 'abnormal' and the greatest incidence (71 %) was recorded in ewes which had been naturally mated. Clearly, uterine insemination was not responsible for such abnormalities, nor did the presence of seminal plasma at or near the site of fertilization affect fertilization or the subsequent development of fertilized eggs.

Multinucleate cells, as observed in Type 2 'abnormal' eggs, represent gross aberrations and such eggs may very well be incapable of full development. However, the low incidence of these eggs—two of 124 examined—suggests that they are of little consequence. Anucleate particles, as observed in Type 1 'abnormal' eggs, may be of little or no importance. The high incidence of this type of egg, particularly in naturally mated ewes, strongly suggests that they are in fact normal in so far as further development is concerned and should be classed as 'atypical' rather than 'abnormal'. Hancock & Hovell (1961) recorded that fertilized sheep eggs with irregular sized blastomeres were capable of full development and Killeen (1969) suggested that eggs similar to those of Type 1 observed in the present study were viable. The low incidence of Type 1 eggs in ewes inseminated with washed semen in Exp. 2 is difficult to explain, particularly as, in Exp. 1, similar treatment resulted in a high incidence of eggs with anucleate particles.

The low proportion of eggs recovered following uterine insemination may indicate the reason for the poor lambing performances recorded following uterine insemination. Overall, uterine insemination gave high fertilization rates in eggs recovered, but the proportion recovered was relatively low. Thus, 20 to 30% less eggs were recovered following uterine insemination than after natural mating in Exp. 2. Surgical interference with the tract seems to result either in expulsion or rapid transport of eggs. Rapid transport would seem to be implicated as the authors (unpublished data) have obtained high recovery rates, as well as high fertilization rates, following uterine insemination when 48 hr, or less, elapsed between insemination and recovery of eggs. In the present study, 60 hr elapsed between insemination and recovery. Thus, it seems that the low lambing performances observed following surgical insemination are due to abnormal transport of eggs resulting from surgical interference.

ACKNOWLEDGMENTS

Grateful acknowledgment for technical assistance is made to Mr A. D. Barnes, Mr R. W. Connors, Mr C. J. Hodges, Mr J. E. McRae, Miss Narelle Flett and Mrs Margaret Jeffery.

Financial support was provided by the Australian Research Grants Committee and the Australian Wool Board. One of us (I.D.K.) was the recipient of a Wool Board Postgraduate Fellowship. PMSG was generously donated by G. D. Searle & Co., Chicago.

REFERENCES

AVERILL, R. L. W. & ROWSON, L. E. A. (1958) Ovum transfer in the sheep. *J. Endocr.* 16, 326.

CHANG, M. C. (1950) The effect of seminal plasma on fertilized rabbit ova. *Proc. natn. Acad. Sci. U.S.A.* 36, 188.

HADEK, R. (1959) Study of the sperm capacitation factor in the genital tract of the female rabbit. *Am. J. vet. Res.* 20, 753.

HANCOCK, J. L. & HOVELL, G. J. R. (1961) Transfer of sheep ova. *J. Reprod. Fert.* 2, 520.

KILLEEN, I. D. (1969) *Studies on fertilization and early development of the ovine ovum.* Ph.D. thesis, University of Sydney.

MATTNER, P. E., ENTWISTLE, K. W. & MARTIN, I. C. A. (1969) Passage, survival and fertility of deep-frozen ram semen in the genital tract of the ewe. *Aust. J. biol. Sci.* 22, 181.

MOORE, N. W. & ROWSON, L. E. A. (1960) Egg transfer in sheep. Factors affecting the survival and development of transferred eggs. *J. Reprod. Fert.* 1, 332.

MOORE, N. W. & SHELTON, J. N. (1964) Egg transfer in sheep. Effect of degree of synchronization between donor and recipient, age of egg, and site of transfer on the survival of transferred eggs. *J. Reprod. Fert.* 7, 145.

SALAMON, S. & LIGHTFOOT, R. J. (1967) Fertilization and embryonic loss in sheep after insemination with deep frozen semen. *Nature, Lond.* 216, 194.

EFFECTS OF SITE OF INSEMINATION, SPERM MOTILITY AND GENITAL TRACT CONTRACTIONS ON TRANSPORT OF SPERMATOZOA IN THE EWE

R. J. LIGHTFOOT AND B. J. RESTALL

INTRODUCTION

The physiological mechanisms responsible for the transport of spermatozoa through the ovine cervix are poorly understood. Starke (1949) and Mattner & Braden (1963) found that spermatozoa can reach the Fallopian tubes within

6 to 8 min of coitus, and such evidence supports the view that contractions of the genital tract account for the passage of spermatozoa through the lower segments. In contrast, the studies of Quinlan, Maré & Roux (1932), Green & Winters (1935), Lopyrin & Loginova (1939) and Dauzier & Wintenberger (1952) indicate that several hours elapse before spermatozoa are found in the Fallopian tubes. Their data suggest that the passage of spermatozoa through the cervix requires approximately 30 min and is effected by the inherent motility of the male gamete.

Because of this conflict, the experiments described herein were designed to examine the relative importance of several factors thought to influence the transport of spermatozoa through the ovine genital tract with particular reference to the cervix.

MATERIALS AND METHODS

Sheep and management

Mature Merino ewes were randomly allocated to treatments on a within-draft basis and inseminated 2 to 16 hr after the onset of oestrus.

Semen

Ejaculates of good initial motility were collected from two mature Merino rams by artificial vagina, pooled and used for insemination without dilution. When required (Exps 2 and 3), spermatozoa were killed (absence of motility, positive nigrosin–eosin staining reaction) by plunging the semen into liquid nitrogen, thawing, and re-freezing.

Technique of insemination

Normal inseminations (external cervical os) were performed with the aid of a duck-billed speculum and headlight. Mucus present in the vagina was removed before insemination. In Exp. 1, the plastic inseminating pipette was inserted as far as possible into the cervix of each ewe and the depth of cervical penetration recorded. In Exps 2 and 3, the pipette was inserted to a uniform depth of approximately 0·5 to 1·0 cm.

A sterile glass pipette with a fine glazed tip was used for inseminations at the level of the internal cervical os (Exp. 3). Following mid-ventral laparotomy under local anaesthesia, the uterus was penetrated just caudal to the internal bifurcation, and the semen deposited near the utero-cervical junction.

In Exps 1 and 2, a dose of 0·1 ml of semen containing 300 to 400×10^6 spermatozoa was used. The inseminate volume was varied in Exp. 3 to allow injection of a constant number of spermatozoa (800×10^6).

Recovery and counting of spermatozoa

The techniques used for recovery and enumeration of spermatozoa from the Fallopian tubes following laparotomy (Exp. 1) and from the Fallopian tubes, uterus and cervix following slaughter by intracardiac injection (Exp. 2), were as described by Lightfoot & Salamon (1970). However, in Exp. 3, after slaughter, the Fallopian tubes and uterus were treated as above, and the cervix was flushed twice with 10 ml of saline from the uterine end. It was then divided into caudal, mid and cranial segments of equal length and the segments were placed in Bouin's fixative. From each segment, transverse sections (6 μm) were cut, mounted, stained (haematoxylin–eosin) and examined microscopically ($\times 400$) for spermatozoa. When large numbers of spermatozoa were present, counting became difficult and so a scoring system (Table 8) was adopted.

Statistical analyses
Data were examined by the appropriate analysis of variance, after transformation according to the function $\log_{10}$ (number of spermatozoa $+2$). Differences between cervical segments (i.e. caudal, mid and cranial) were examined by the procedure for split-plot experiments (Cochran & Cox, 1957).

EXPERIMENTAL DESIGN AND RESULTS

Experiment 1: *The effects of oxytocin and depth of insemination on the number of spermatozoa in the Fallopian tubes 2 hr after insemination*

Three groups each consisting of twenty ewes received either 0, 1·0 or 10·0 i.u. of oxytocin (Syntocinon, intramuscularly) at the time of insemination. Spermatozoa were recovered by flushing the Fallopian tubes *in vivo* 2 hr after insemination.

TABLE 1

EXP. 1. THE EFFECTS OF OXYTOCIN AND DEPTH OF INSEMINATION ON THE NUMBER OF SPERMATOZOA RECOVERED FROM THE FALLOPIAN TUBES 2 HR AFTER INSEMINATION

Treatment	No. of ewes examined	No. of ewes yielding sperm.	Mean no. of sperm.
Dose of oxytocin (i.u.)			
0	20	7	1948
1	20	5	71
10	20	2	2
Depth of insemination			
Shallow: < 1 cm	32	6	34
Medium: 1 to 3 cm	21	4	35
Deep: > 3 cm	7	4	5520
Overall	60	14	674

Only fourteen (23%) of the sixty ewes examined yielded spermatozoa (Table 1). Of the ewes receiving either 0, 1·0 or 10·0 i.u. oxytocin, spermatozoa were recovered from 35, 25 and 10% respectively (0 versus 1·0 and 10·0 i.u., $\chi_1^2 = 2\cdot28$, $0\cdot1 < P < 0\cdot2$). The administration of oxytocin also depressed the mean numbers of spermatozoa recovered.

Both the proportion of ewes yielding spermatozoa (57% versus 19%; $\chi_1^2 = 3\cdot17$, $0\cdot05 < P < 0\cdot1$) and the mean number of spermatozoa recovered

TABLE 2

EXP. 2A. THE EFFECTS OF SPERM MOTILITY, HALOTHANE ANAESTHESIA AND OXYTOCIN ON THE NUMBERS OF SPERMATOZOA RECOVERED FROM THE CERVIX, UTERUS AND FALLOPIAN TUBES OF EWES SLAUGHTERED 30 MIN AFTER INSEMINATION

Treatment no.	Treatment			No. of ewes	Cervix			Uterus	Fallopian tubes
	Sperm motility	Anaesthesia	Oxytocin		Caudal	Mid	Cranial	Mean no. of sperm	Mean no. of sperm
					$10^{-3} \times$ Mean no. of sperm				
1	+	−	−	8	4678 *6·368* (8)	171 *4·243* (8)	165 *2·977* (6)	1604 (2)	17 (2)
2	+	−	+	8	6904 *6·736* (8)	484 *4·950* (8)	10 *3·344* (7)	18 (1)	15 (2)
3	+	+	−	8	7823 *6·538* (8)	569 *3·929* (7)	11 *3·193* (7)	256 (2)	9 (1)
4	+	+	+	9	6417 *6·544* (8)	801 *5·192* (8)	6 *3·111* (7)	19 (2)	39 (2)
5	−	−	−	8	1598 *4·772* (8)	9 *2·903* (6)	10 *2·082* (4)	331 (2)	52 (2)
6	−	−	+	8	151 *4·640* (8)	2 *1·783* (4)	23 *2·137* (4)	0 (0)	62 (2)
7	−	+	−	8	935 *5·068* (8)	2 *1·462* (3)	1 *0·717* (1)	18 (2)	0 (0)
8	−	+	+	8	527 *5·076* (8)	1 *1·474* (3)	1 *1·459* (3)	27 (2)	0 (0)

Logarithmic means in italics. The number of ewes yielding spermatozoa are shown in parentheses.

93

(5520 versus 34) were higher for the ewes in which semen could be deposited further than 3 cm into the cervix.

Experiment 2A: The effects of sperm motility and contractions of the genital tract on the distribution of spermatozoa throughout the genital tract 30 min after insemination
A $2 \times 2 \times 2$ factorial design (n = 8, N = 64) was used to examine the following factors:

(1) Sperm motility — Live versus dead spermatozoa
(2) Inhibition of genital tract contractions — Nil versus halothane anaesthesia
(3) Stimulation of genital tract contractions — Nil versus oxytocin

TABLE 3

EXP. 2A. SUMMARY OF ANALYSIS OF VARIANCE FOR NUMBERS OF SPERMATOZOA RECOVERED FROM THE CERVIX

Source of variation		d.f.	Variance ratio
Sperm motility	(A)	1	69·20***
Halothane anaesthesia	(B)	1	1·25
Oxytocin	(C)	1	0·60
A × B		1	1·09
A × C		1	1·17
B × C		1	0·36
A × B × C		1	0·61
Error 1 (Ewes within A × B × C)		56	2·67†
Cervical segment	(D)		
Linear		1	252·87***
Quadratic		1	19·61***
A × D			
A × linear		1	0·06
A × quadratic		1	8·58**
Pooled (non-significant) first, second and third order interactions		12	1·11
Error 2		112	1·41†

** $P < 0.01$;   *** $P < 0.001$.
† Error mean square.

The effects of halothane anaesthesia and oxytocin on spontaneous contractions of the oestrous ovine genital tract *in vivo* have been evaluated by Lightfoot (1970a, b). Halothane anaesthesia resulted in complete inhibition of cervical and uterine contractions in 79% and 43%, respectively, of the ewes examined, but slight residual activity was evident in the remaining cases. The inhibition was not overcome by vaginal stimulation, but oxytocin (800 mU, intravenously) produced a contractile response of lesser intensity and duration than that recorded in conscious ewes.

In the present experiment, the relevant ewes were inseminated approximately 5 min after establishing anaesthesia (surgical level) and killed while still

TABLE 4

EXP. 2A. EFFECTS OF SPERM MOTILITY, HALOTHANE ANAESTHESIA AND OXYTOCIN ON THE NUMBERS OF SPERMATOZOA RECOVERED FROM THE CERVIX, UTERUS AND FALLOPIAN TUBES OF EWES SLAUGHTERED 30 MIN AFTER INSEMINATION

Treatment	No. of ewes	Cervix			Uterus	Fallopian tubes
		Caudal $10^{-3} \times$ mean	Mid no.	Cranial of sperm.	Mean no. of sperm.	Mean no. of sperm.
Sperm motility +	32	6·455 *6·547* (32)	507 *4·579* (31)	48 *3·156* (27)	474 (7)	20 (7)
−	32	803 *4·889* (32)	3 *1·905* (16)	9 *1·599* (12)	94 (6)	28 (4)
Halothane anaesthesia −	32	3333 *5·629* (32)	166 *3·470* (26)	52 *2·635* (21)	488 (5)	36 (8)
+	32	3926 *5·807* (32)	343 *3·014* (21)	5 *2·120* (18)	80 (8)	12 (3)
Oxytocin −	32	3759 *5·687* (32)	188 *3·134* (24)	46 *2·242* (18)	552 (8)	19 (5)
+	32	3500 *5·749* (32)	322 *3·350* (23)	10 *2·513* (21)	16 (5)	29 (6)
Overall	64	3629 *5·718* (64)	255 *3·242* (47)	28 *2·377* (39)	284 (13)	24 (11)

Logarithmic mean in italics. The number of ewes yielding spermatozoa are shown in parentheses.

TABLE 5

EXP. 2A. EFFECT OF HALOTHANE ANAESTHESIA ON THE NUMBERS OF SPERMATOZOA RECOVERED FROM THE CERVIX, UTERUS AND FALLOPIAN TUBES OF EWES SLAUGHTERED 30 MIN AFTER INSEMINATION WITH IMMOTILE SPERMATOZOA (TREATMENTS 5 TO 8 IN TABLE 2)

Treatment	No. of ewes*	Cervix			Uterus	Fallopian tubes
		Caudal $10^{-3} \times$ Mean	Mid no.	Cranial of sperm.	Mean no. of sperm.	Mean no. of sperm.
Conscious ewes	16	875 *4·706* (16)	5 *2·343* (10)	16 *2·110* (8)	166 (2)	57 (4)
Anaesthetized ewes	16	731 *5·072* (16)	1 *1·468* (6)	1 *1·088* (4)	23 (4)	0 (0)

Logarithmic means in italics. The number of ewes yielding spermatozoa are shown in parentheses.

* Oxytocin treatments pooled.

under anaesthesia. Oxytocin (Syntocinon, 1·0 i.u. in 1 ml) was injected intravenously 1 min before, and again 15 min after insemination. All ewes were slaughtered 30 min after insemination and the various parts of the genital tract were ligated within 3 min of slaughter.

Marked differences in the position and activity of the genital tracts were observed at slaughter. Halothane anaesthesia, without oxytocin, resulted in complete relaxation of the tract and the absence of spontaneous contractions. In contrast, uteri in conscious ewes that received oxytocin lay in the high-retracted position and exhibited pronounced contractile activity.

The effects of all treatments on the numbers of spermatozoa recovered from the genital tract are shown in Table 2, the relevant analysis of variance in Table 3 and treatment main effects in Table 4.

Cervix. Of the three factors examined, only sperm motility had a significant effect $(P < 0.001)$ on the mean number of spermatozoa recovered from the cervix. Few spermatozoa were found after insemination with immotile, compared with motile, cells (Table 4).

Split-plot analysis (Table 3) revealed a significant interaction $(P < 0.01)$ due to an effect of sperm motility on the relative numbers of spermatozoa recovered from adjacent cervical segments. Insemination with motile cells led to an almost linear reduction in the number recovered from successively ascending segments, whereas the use of immotile cells resulted in a steep fall in sperm numbers between the caudal and mid regions, with little further reduction in the cranial segment.

Following insemination with immotile spermatozoa, but not with motile cells, halothane anaesthesia inhibited the progression of spermatozoa through the cervix (Table 5).

Analysis of the data for inseminations with immotile spermatozoa only, showed that the interaction was significant (halothane anaesthesia × cervical segment, linear; $P < 0.05$).

Of the thirty-two ewes inseminated with immotile cells, all animals, both conscious and anaesthetized, yielded spermatozoa from the caudal segment of the cervix. In the mid-cervical segment, however, anaesthesia reduced the proportion of ewes yielding spermatozoa from 63% to 38%, and in the cranial segment, from 50% to 25%.

Uterus and Fallopian tubes. Spermatozoa were recovered from the uterine flushings in only thirteen (20%) of the sixty-four ewes examined. The results (Tables 2, 4 and 5) suggest that among ewes in which transport occurred, the quantitative passage of spermatozoa to the uterus was depressed by halothane anaesthesia, by injections of oxytocin, and by insemination with immotile spermatozoa.

Spermatozoa were found in tubal flushings from only eleven (17%) of the sixty-four ewes and there were no obvious differences between any of the treatment main effects shown in Table 4. Examination of the data for inseminations with immotile cells only, however, revealed that no spermatozoa were recovered from the Fallopian tubes of the sixteen anaesthetized ewes, whereas a mean of 226 tubal spermatozoa were recovered from four of the conscious animals (Table 5).

Experiment 2B: *The effects of natural service versus artificial insemination on the distribution of spermatozoa throughout the genital tract 30 min after semen deposition*

In order to compare sperm transport following natural service with that resulting from artificial insemination in the control treatment (live spermatozoa, no anaesthesia, no oxytocin) of the main experiment (2A), an additional eight ewes from the same flock were allowed one natural service with a ram and slaughtered 30 min later. The ewes were allocated to the natural service treatment during the conduct of the main experiment and successive ewes were served by either one of the two rams on an alternate basis.

TABLE 6

EXP. 2B. EFFECT OF ARTIFICIAL INSEMINATION VERSUS NATURAL SERVICE ON THE NUMBERS OF SPERMATOZOA RECOVERED FROM THE CERVIX, UTERUS AND FALLOPIAN TUBES 30 MIN AFTER SEMEN DEPOSITION

Method of insemination	No. of ewes	Cervix			Uterus	Fallopian tubes
		Caudal	Mid	Cranial	Mean no. of sperm.	Mean no. of sperm.
		$10^{-3} \times$	Mean no.	of sperm.		
Artificial insemination	8*	4678 *6·368* (8)	171 *4·243* (8)	165 *2·977* (6)	1604 (2)	17 (2)
Natural service	8	22714 *7·001* (8)	1120 *5·471* (8)	281 *4·485* (8)	406 (2)	45 (5)

Logarithmic means in italics. The number of ewes yielding spermatozoa are shown in parentheses.

* Ewes from Treatment 1, Exp. 2A (Table 2).

Significantly more spermatozoa ($P < 0·05$) were recovered from the cervix of ewes following natural service than following artificial insemination (Table 6); similar numbers of spermatozoa were found in the uterus for both treatments; however, more ewes yielded tubal spermatozoa following natural service.

Experiment 3: *The effects of site of insemination and sperm motility on the distribution of spermatozoa throughout the genital tract 2 hr after insemination*

The experiment was of factorial design (2×2, $n = 11$, $N = 44$) and examined the effects of site of insemination (external cervical os versus internal cervical os) and sperm motility (live versus dead spermatozoa) on the distribution of spermatozoa throughout the genital tract 2 hr after insemination.

Spermatozoa in flushings from the tract. The mean number of spermatozoa recovered per ewe was approximately 119×10^6 or 15% of the 800×10^6 inseminated. Most of this difference may be attributed to expulsion and/or drainage of mucus and spermatozoa from the vagina between insemination and slaughter as reported by Conley & Hawk (1969). Phagocytosis of spermatozoa, and incomplete recovery during flushing, would also have contributed to the loss.

The results (Table 7) show that the numbers of spermatozoa recovered from the vagina 2 hr after insemination were independent of both sperm motility and site of insemination, but the numbers of spermatozoa recovered from the cervix were strongly influenced by these factors. Semen deposition at the uterine end of the cervix resulted in higher numbers than normal insemination ($P < 0.001$) and motile spermatozoa were more effective than immotile cells ($P < 0.01$). The data suggest that following insemination at the level of the external cervical os, motile spermatozoa were more effective in entering the cervix, whereas after insemination at the level of the internal cervical os, large numbers of both motile and immotile spermatozoa entered and traversed the cervix in the caudal direction. However, the motile cells were more effectively retained within the lumen of the cervix.

TABLE 7

EXP. 3. THE EFFECTS OF SITE OF INSEMINATION AND SPERM MOTILITY ON THE DISTRIBUTION OF SPERMATOZOA IN THE GENITAL TRACT 2 HR AFTER INSEMINATION

Site of insemination	Sperm motility	No. of ewes	Vagina	Cervix	Uterus	Fallopian tubes
				$10^{-3} \times$ Mean no. of sperm.		
External cervical os	+	11	105206 *7.909*	2919 *6.064*	6 *2.581*	0.604 *1.920*
	−	11	135318 *8.027*	846 *5.358*	2 *1.606*	0.499 *1.177*
Internal cervical os	+	11	114460 *7.156*	22746 *7.138*	7373 *6.281*	71.367 *4.516*
	−	11	74642 *7.298*	3094 *6.196*	5226 *6.003*	5.875 *2.860*

Logarithmic means in italics.

Many more spermatozoa were found in uterine flushings following semen deposition at the internal cervical os than after normal insemination ($P < 0.001$). Only 5 to 7×10^6 of the 800×10^6 spermatozoa that were deposited at the utero-cervical junction remained in the uterus and of the total spermatozoa recovered from the tract, approximately 80% had passed caudally to the vagina.

Results for the Fallopian tubes were similar to those for the cervix in that both insemination at the internal cervical os ($P < 0.001$) and the use of motile cells ($P < 0.01$) resulted in significantly more spermatozoa being recovered. Spermatozoa were found in the Fallopian tubes of seven and four of the eleven ewes in each treatment following normal insemination with motile and immotile spermatozoa respectively. Only one ewe (inseminated with immotile cells) failed to yield spermatozoa in the tubal flushings following semen deposition at the internal cervical os. There were no significant interactions.

Spermatozoa in the cervical sections. Results for the numbers of spermatozoa observed in transverse sections from the caudal, mid and cranial regions of the cervix (after flushing) are presented in Table 8. When immotile cells were used, no spermatozoa were found between the mucosal folds following insemination at the external os, and only very low numbers after insemination at the utero-cervical junction. Consequently, an analysis of variance was performed on the data pertaining to inseminations with motile cells only. In this case, large numbers of spermatozoa were observed in the cervical sections, particularly after semen deposition at the utero-cervical junction ($P < 0.01$). With both methods of insemination, the numbers of spermatozoa fell from the caudal to the cranial end of the cervix but the rate of decline was steeper following semen deposition at the external cervical os (site of insemination × position in cervix, linear; $P < 0.01$).

TABLE 8

EXP. 3. THE EFFECTS OF SITE OF INSEMINATION AND SPERM MOTILITY ON THE NUMBERS OF SPERMATOZOA COUNTED IN TRANSVERSE SECTIONS CUT FROM THE CAUDAL, MID AND CRANIAL SEGMENTS OF THE CERVIX AFTER FLUSHING

Site of insemination	Sperm motility	Cervix			Total
		Caudal	Mid	Cranial	
External cervical os	+	3·18	2·27	0·73	6·18
	−	0·00	0·00	0·00	0·00
Internal cervical os	+	3·55	2·91	2·82	9·28
	−	0·36	0·00	0·27	0·63

The data are mean classification scores (see below) from eleven ewes/treatment.

No. of spermatozoa counted in sections	Classification score
0	0
1 to 9	1
10 to 99	2
100 to 999	3
⩾ 1000	4

DISCUSSION

In general, the results of the experiments reported here support the findings of Phillips & Andrews (1937), Schott & Phillips (1941), Starke (1949), Mattner & Braden (1963) and Mattner (1963a) that spermatozoa can reach the Fallopian tubes of the ewe within 30 min of their deposition in, or near, the external cervical os. The results do not agree with reports by Quinlan et al. (1932), Green & Winters (1935), Kelley (1937), Lopyrin & Loginova (1939), Dauzier & Wintenberger (1952), Dauzier (1958) and Edgar & Asdell (1960) which suggest that several hours usually elapse before spermatozoa can be found in the Fallopian tubes. Apart from obvious differences in techniques used for detecting spermatozoa, the conflicting results could be due to the fact that rapid transport occurs only in a proportion of ewes and the proportion may be lower following artificial insemination than natural service. Rapid transport was evident in only 25% of the (control treatment) ewes in Exp. 2A, and in no more than 13% of the ewes studied by Lightfoot & Salamon (1970). Even after 2 hr, spermatozoa were found in the tubes of only 35% and 64% of the control ewes examined in Exps 1 and 3 respectively and the numbers of cells recovered were highly variable and often quite low.

Regardless of the occurrence or failure of rapid transport, there can be little doubt from Exps 2 and 3 that sperm motility is an essential prerequisite for the quantitative distribution of spermatozoa throughout the genital tract. Active sperm-tail flagellation was important for the initial entry of large numbers of spermatozoa into the cervix and their progression in reasonable numbers to the mid and cranial segments. In addition, the results of Exp. 3 have shown that motility is required for spermatozoa to penetrate between the deeply divided mucosal folds of the cervix. Immotile spermatozoa did not penetrate as they were easily removed by flushing, confirming the recent observation of Mattner & Braden (1969). Thus, the formation and retention of the sperm reservoir in the ovine cervix is primarily dependent on the motility of the spermatozoon—a view in accord with the conclusions of Mattner (1966).

The evidence suggesting participation of vaginal, cervical and/or uterine contractions in the transport of spermatozoa through the ovine cervix is well documented by Mattner & Braden (1963) and Mattner (1963b) but their observations on the transport of immotile particles are in conflict with those of Dauzier (1953). The present results (Exps 2 and 3) show quite clearly that, at least in a proportion of ewes, low numbers of immotile spermatozoa can ascend through the cervix. Further, as immotile spermatozoa do not penetrate between the mucosal folds, it can be assumed that they pass through the cervix mainly by way of the central lumen of the canal where presumably a more fluid environment exists due to the caudal drainage of uterine secretions. Uterine and/or cervical contractions appear to be responsible for this phase of sperm transport as inhibition of the contractile activity of the genital tract by halothane anaesthesia significantly reduced the number of spermatozoa recovered from the mid and cranial regions of the cervix.

Participation of uterine contractions in the movement of spermatozoa from the uterus to the Fallopian tubes, even though sperm motility appeared to be quantitatively more important, was supported by the results of Exp. 3. Considerable numbers of immotile spermatozoa were recovered from the Fallopian tubes 2 hr after their deposition at the utero-cervical junction. This observation confirms findings of a similar nature reported previously by Dauzier (1958) and Mattner (1963b). Some caution is necessary in the interpretation of experiments involving uterine insemination, however, as the technique may stimulate an abnormal pattern of uterine contractions possibly due either to physical manipulation of the uterus or to the action of pharmacologically active substances that occur in ram semen, such as prostaglandins. Nevertheless, additional evidence that myometrial activity supplements sperm motility in this phase of transport is seen in the results of Exp. 2A. Following cervical insemination with immotile cells, no spermatozoa were found in tubal flushings from anaesthetized ewes, whereas several conscious ewes yielded tubal spermatozoa (Table 5).

The effects of administering oxytocin on the movement of spermatozoa or inert material through the female reproductive tract have been studied in several species and the subject has been discussed in reviews by Cross (1959)

100

and Fitzpatrick (1966). Evidence in the sheep, however, is limited, but reports by Thibault & Wintenberger-Torres (1967) and Lang & Oh (1968) do not support the concept that oxytocin hastens the ascent of spermatozoa through the ewe's reproductive tract. The results of Exps 1 and 2A reported here, further indicate that, although low doses appear to have little effect, high doses of oxytocin in the oestrous ewe are detrimental to the transport of spermatozoa through the genital tract. Similarly, low doses of oxytocin administered at the time of insemination appear to have little effect on fertility in the ewe (Jones, 1968; Jones, Martin & Lapwood, 1969; Salamon & Lightfoot, 1970) but high doses (5 to 20 i.u.) reduce both fertilization (Lightfoot & Salamon, 1970) and lambing rates (Salamon & Lightfoot, 1970).

In conclusion, the present study indicates that, although contractions of the ovine genital tract supplement sperm motility in effecting transport of spermatozoa through the uterus and, to a lesser extent, the cervix, active flagellation oy the sperm-tail appears essential for the establishment of the cervical population of spermatozoa and their subsequent distribution throughout the uterus and Fallopian tubes in physiological numbers.

ACKNOWLEDGMENTS

We are indebted to Professor T. J. Robinson and Dr S. Salamon, Department of Animal Husbandry, University of Sydney, and to Professor C. W. Emmens, Department of Veterinary Physiology, University of Sydney, for their interest and criticisms. Syntocinon was generously donated by Sandoz, Australia Pty Ltd. This work was supported in part by grants from the Australian Research Grants Committee and the Australian Wool Board.

REFERENCES

COCHRAN, W. G. & COX, G. M. (1957) *Experimental designs*, 2nd edn. John Wiley, New York.

CONLEY, H. H. & HAWK, H. W. (1969) Loss of spermatozoa from reproductive tracts of ewes. *J. Anim. Sci.* 29, 186.

CROSS, B. A. (1959) *Hypothalamic influences on sperm transport in the male and female genital tract.* In: Endocrinology of Reproduction, p. 167. Ed. C. W. Lloyd. Academic Press, New York.

DAUZIER, L. (1953) Recherches sur les facteurs de la remontée des spermatozoïdes dans les voies génitales femelles. Étude chez la brebis (col de l'utérus). *C. r. Séanc. Soc. Biol.* 147, 1556.

DAUZIER, L. (1958) Physiologie du déplacement des spermatozoïdes dans les voies génitales femelles chez la brebis et la vache. *Annls Zootech.* 7, 281.

DAUZIER, L. & WINTENBERGER, S. (1952) Recherches sur la fécondation chez les mammifères: la remontée des spermatozoïdes dans le tractus génital de la brebis. *C. r. Séanc. Soc. Biol.* 146, 67.

EDGAR, D. G. & ASDELL, S. A. (1960) Spermatozoa in the female genital tract. *J. Endocr.* 21, 321.

FITZPATRICK, R. J. (1966). *The posterior pituitary gland and the female reproductive tract.* In: The Pituitary Gland, Vol. III, p. 453. Eds. G. W. Harris and B. T. Donovan. Butterworths, London.

GREEN, W. W. & WINTERS, L. M. (1935) Studies on the physiology of reproduction in the sheep. III. The time of ovulation and the rate of sperm travel. *Anat. Rec.* 61, 457.

JONES, R. C. (1968) The fertility of ewes injected with synthetic oxytocin following artificial insemination. *Aust. Jnl exp. Agric. & Anim. Husb.* 8, 13.

JONES, R. C., MARTIN, I. C. A. & LAPWOOD, K. R. (1969) Studies of the artificial insemination of sheep: the effects on fertility of diluting ram semen, stage of oestrus of the ewe at insemination, and injection of synthetic oxytocin. *Aust. J. agric. Res.* 20, 141.

KELLEY, R. B. (1937) Studies in fertility of sheep. *Bull. Coun. scient. ind. Res., Melb.* No. 112.

LANG, D. R. & OH, K. Y. (1968) Distribution of spermatozoa in the reproductive tract of the Romney ewe. *Proc. N.Z. Soc. Anim. Prod.* 28, 120.

LIGHTFOOT, R. J. (1970a) *Studies of factors affecting the survival, physiological transport and fertility of ram spermatozoa after freezing by the pellet method*. Ph.D. thesis, University of Sydney.

LIGHTFOOT, R. J. (1970b) The contractile activity of the genital tract of the ewe in response to oxytocin and mating. *J. Reprod. Fert.* **21,** 376.

LIGHTFOOT, R. J. & SALAMON, S. (1970) The fertility of ram spermatozoa frozen by the pellet method. I. Transport and viability of spermatozoa within the genital tract of the ewe. *J. Reprod. Fert.* **22,** 385.

LOPYRIN, A. I. & LOGINOVA, N. V. (1939) Rate of movement and time of survival of spermatozoa in the genital tract of the ewe. *Sov. Zootekh.* No. 2/3, 144. (*Anim. Breed. Abstr.* **8,** 256.)

MATTNER, P. E. (1963a) Spermatozoa in the genital tract of the ewe. II. Distribution after coitus. *Aust. J. biol. Sci.* **16,** 688.

MATTNER, P. E. (1963b) Spermatozoa in the genital tract of the ewe. III. The role of spermatozoan motility and of uterine contractions in transport of spermatozoa. *Aust. J. biol. Sci.* **16,** 877.

MATTNER, P. E. (1966) Formation and retention of the spermatozoan reservoir in the cervix of the ruminant. *Nature, Lond.* **212,** 1479.

MATTNER, P. E. & BRADEN, A. W. H. (1963) Spermatozoa in the genital tract of the ewe. I. Rapidity of transport. *Aust. J. biol. Sci.* **16,** 473.

MATTNER, P. E. & BRADEN, A. W. H. (1969) Comparison of the distribution of motile and immotile spermatozoa in the ovine cervix. *Aust. J. biol. Sci.* **22,** 1069.

PHILLIPS, R. W. & ANDREWS, F. N. (1937) The speed of travel of ram spermatozoa. *Anat. Rec.* **68,** 127.

QUINLAN, J., MARÉ, G. S. & ROUX, L. L. (1932) The vitality of the spermatozoon in the genital tract of the Merino ewe, with special reference to its practical application in breeding. *Rep. vet. Res. Un. S. Afr.* No. **18,** 831.

SALAMON S. & LIGHTFOOT, R. J. (1970) The fertility of ram spermatozoa frozen by the pellet method. III. The effects of insemination technique, oxytocin and relaxin on lambing. *J. Reprod. Fert.* **22,** 409.

SCHOTT, R. G. & PHILLIPS, R. W. (1941) The rate of sperm travel and time of ovulation in sheep. *Anat. Rec.* **79,** 531.

STARKE, N. C. (1949) The sperm picture of rams of different breeds as an indication of their fertility. II. The rate of sperm travel in the genital tract of the ewe. *Onderstepoort J. vet. Sci. Anim. Ind.* **22,** 415.

THIBAULT, C. & WINTENBERGER-TORRES, S. (1967) Oxytocin and sperm transport in the ewe. *Int. J. Fert.* **12,** 410.

TRANSPORT OF SPERMATOZOA, AND FERTILIZATION IN THE EWE FOLLOWING CERVICAL AND UTERINE INSEMINATION EARLY AND LATE IN OESTRUS

By I. D. Killeen and N. W. Moore

I. Introduction

In the ewe high fertilization rates can be achieved by depositing semen directly into the uterine horns or fallopian tubes as late as 48 hr after the onset of oestrus, but cervical insemination carried out 36 or more hours after the onset of oestrus results in complete failure of fertilization (Killeen and Moore 1970). Similarly, Mattner and Braden (1969) reported poor fertilization in ewes cervically inseminated late in oestrus and this was associated with lowered numbers of spermatozoa in the cervix, uterus, and tubes.

Killeen and Moore (1970) reported a marked effect of site of insemination on the relationships between fertilization and lambing performance. Whilst no eggs were fertilized and no ewes lambed to cervical insemination at 36 or 48 hr after the onset of oestrus, 13 of 24 ewes inseminated into the uterus at similar times after oestrus had fertilized eggs, but only 1 of 24 lambed. Whole semen was used for insemination and thus with uterine inseminations there was a distinct chance of close contact between recently ovulated eggs and seminal plasma, a component of semen which in the rabbit has a deleterious effect upon the viability of fertilized eggs (Chang 1950; Hadek 1959). With cervical insemination the plasma components of semen are probably lost, or at least diluted, during passage through the genital tract.

103

The present experiment was designed first to examine the effect of time and site of insemination on transport of spermatozoa and on fertilization; and second, to study the part played by seminal plasma in transport of spermatozoa, fertilization, and early development of fertilized eggs.

II. MATERIALS AND METHODS

(a) Experimental Animals and Design

A flock of 250 mature cyclic Merino ewes, 10 vasectomized rams, and 6 entire Merino rams of proven fertility were available for the experiment. The ewes were run continuously with the vasectomized rams and they were inspected for oestrus twice daily (0600 and 1800 hr). In all, 192 ewes were included in an experiment of the following design:

(1) Site of insemination—uterus v. cervix;

(2) Treatment of semen—none v. diluted 1 : 2 v. seminal plasma removed;

(3) Time of insemination (hours after onset of oestrus)—0 v. 24;

(4) Time of recovery of spermatozoa and eggs (hours after insemination)—6 v. 24.

Factorial: $2 \times 3 \times 2 \times 2$; $n = 8$; $N = 192$.

(b) Insemination

Inseminations were made into the cervix or the tip of both uterine horns immediately, or 24 hr after, the ewes were first detected in oestrus (i.e. 0–12 and 24–36 hr after the onset of oestrus). Uterine inseminations were carried out under local anaesthesia (Xylocaine).

(c) Treatment of Semen

Pooled semen collected by artificial vagina from at least three rams was inseminated as freshly ejaculated semen, or diluted 1 : 2 with normal saline and then inseminated, or inseminated after removal of the seminal plasma. Seminal plasma was removed by repeated washing and centrifugation. A volume of $9 \cdot 5$ ml normal saline was added to $0 \cdot 5$ ml freshly ejaculated semen and then centrifuged for 10 min (300–400 g). After centrifuging $9 \cdot 0$ ml of the supernatant was removed and replaced by a similar volume of normal saline. The spermatozoa were resuspended by vigorous shaking and the process of centrifuging and removal of supernatant was repeated a further five times. The calculated final concentration of seminal plasma was less than 1 part in 2×10^6.

Prior to insemination the concentration of spermatozoa and the proportion of "live" spermatozoa in each sample of semen were estimated and the estimates were used to adjust the volume of inseminate so that each ewe received $30–40 \times 10^7$ live spermatozoa (cervical inseminations) or $3–4 \times 10^7$ live spermatozoa per horn (uterine inseminations). The concentration of spermatozoa was estimated by haemocytometer counts, and the proportion of live spermatozoa was estimated by staining with a mixture of nigrosin and eosin (Hancock 1952). The volume of inseminate varied from $0 \cdot 10–0 \cdot 60$ ml (cervix) or $0 \cdot 01–0 \cdot 06$ ml (uterine horn).

(d) Recovery of Spermatozoa and Eggs

Eggs and spermatozoa were recovered by flushing each fallopian tube with 2 ml normal saline whilst the ewes were under general anaesthesia (Nembutal). The flushings were collected in large-mouthed collecting bowls and eggs were removed from the bowls in a minimal volume of fluid. The flushings were then transferred to a glass tube, the bowls washed with 1 ml saline, and the washings added to the tube.

Eggs were examined before and after staining with 1% orcein. Normal cleavage and penetration or activation by spermatozoa of uncleaved eggs were used as the criteria of fertilization.

(e) Estimation of the Numbers of Spermatozoa

The method used for estimating the numbers of spermatozoa in the tubal flushings was similar to that described by Quinlivan and Robinson (1967). Each sample was distributed evenly over six standard microscope slides (3 by 1 in.), a coverslip (22 by 40 mm), "pillared" on Vaseline, was gently lowered onto the slides, and the number of spermatozoa in one lengthwise traverse on each slide was recorded ($\times 400$ magnification using phase-contrast). One spermatozoa in six traverses represented a total of 48 spermatozoa in the complete flushings.

(f) Statistical Procedures

Standard analyses of variance and tests of χ^2 were applied to the primary or appropriately transformed data. The complete absence of spermatozoa in some flushings and the skewed nature of the distribution of number of spermatozoa found in individual flushings made transformation of the primary data imperative. Standard analyses of variance were used after $\log_{10}(x+1)$ transformation of this data.

III. Results

(a) Recovery and Fertilization of Eggs

No ewe inseminated at 0 hr after the detection of oestrus and laparotomized 6 hr later had ovulated at the time of laparotomy, and a further 16 ewes inseminated at 0 hr and laparotomized 24 hr later had not ovulated at laparotomy (Table 1).

TABLE 1

RECOVERY AND FERTILIZATION OF EGGS FOLLOWING UTERINE AND CERVICAL INSEMINATION AT 0 AND 24 HR AFTER THE DETECTION OF OESTRUS

Data pooled for treatment of semen

Time of Insemination (hr)*	Time of Recovery (hr)*	No. of Ewes Insemin-ated	No. of Ewes Flushed†	No. which Yielded Eggs	No. which Yielded Fertilized Eggs
Cervical insemination					
0	6	24	0	—	—
	24	24	16	12(75%)‡	8(73%)
24	30	24	24	23(96%)	0(0%)
	48	24	24	21(88%)	8(38%)
Total		96	64	56(88%)	16(29%)
Uterine insemination					
0	6	24	0	—	—
	24	24	16	14(88%)‡	9(69%)
24	30	24	24	16(67%)‡	11(73%)
	48	24	24	18(75%)	18(100%)
Total		96	64	48(75%)	38(83%)
Grand total		192	128	104(81%)	54(53%)

* Hours after detection of oestrus.

† Ewes that had ovulated at the time of recovery.

‡ One ewe in each group with fractured egg—no fertilization data available.

Eggs were recovered from 104 of the 128 ewes which had ovulated. Two eggs were recovered from three of five ewes which had two ovulations and in all three ewes both eggs were fertilized. The remaining ewes were monovular. Site of insemination had no effect on recovery of eggs, nor was there any overall effect of time of insemination. However, in ewes which were inseminated at 24 hr the proportion of ewes which yielded eggs following uterine insemination was less than that following cervical insemination (34 of 48 v. 44 of 48; $\chi_1^2 = 5\cdot54$; $P < 0\cdot02$).

Fractured eggs from which the ooplasm had escaped were recovered from three ewes and no fertilization data were available on these animals. Thus, fertilized eggs were recovered from 54 of 101 ewes. There was no effect of treatment of semen on the proportion of ewes with fertilized eggs, but there was a major effect of site of insemination due to very poor fertilization in ewes cervically inseminated 24 hr after the detection of oestrus (16 of 55 v. 38 of 46 ewes fertile; $\chi_1^2 = 26 \cdot 72$; $P < 0 \cdot 001$). Following insemination at 24 hr, irrespective of site of insemination, the proportion of ewes which had fertilized eggs tended to increase when the time elapsing between insemination and recovery was increased from 6 to 24 hr (cervical: 0 of 23 v. 8 of 21 ewes; $\chi_1^2 = 8 \cdot 30$; $P < 0 \cdot 01$; uterine: 11 of 15 v. 18 of 18 ewes; $\chi_1^2 = 3 \cdot 30$; $0 \cdot 10 > P > 0 \cdot 05$).

TABLE 2

NUMBER OF EWES WITH SPERMATOZOA AND ESTIMATES OF MEAN NUMBERS OF SPERMATOZOA RECOVERED FROM THE FALLOPIAN TUBES AFTER CERVICAL AND UTERINE INSEMINATION AT 0 AND 24 HR AFTER THE DETECTION OF OESTRUS

Main effects

Main Effect	No. of Ewes with Spermatozoa		Estimated Mean No. of Spermatozoa Recovered	
	Cervix*	Uterus*	Cervix*	Uterus*
1. Time of insemination ($n = 48$)				
0 hr†	39	48	2,300	28,200
24 hr†	21	48	600	19,900
Significance of difference	< 0:001	n.s.	< 0·001	< 0·05
2. Time of flushing ($n = 48$)				
6 hr‡	25	48	200	23,000
24 hr‡	35	48	2,700	25,100
Significance of difference	< 0·05	n.s.	< 0·001	n.s.
3. Treatment of semen ($n = 32$)				
Nil	25	32	1,600	21,600
Diluted 1 : 2	16	32	1,700	24,800
Fully washed	19	32	900	25,700
Significance of difference	< 0·05	n.s.	n.s.	n.s.
Total ($n = 96$)	60	96	1,500	24,100

* Site of insemination.　　† Hours after detection of oestrus.　　‡ Hours after insemination.

Only 7 of the 47 unfertilized eggs that were recovered had spermatozoa attached to their zonae pellucidae. Gross abnormalities of fertilization were shown by 11 fertilized eggs. Nine were polyspermic and two were digynic. All except one of the abnormal eggs were recovered following uterine insemination, but the incidence of abnormal eggs was not affected by treatment of semen or time of insemination.

(b) Recovery of Spermatozoa

Spermatozoa were recovered from the fallopian tubes of all ewes after uterine insemination, whereas no spermatozoa were found in the flushings of 36 of the 96 ewes inseminated cervically (Table 2). Within cervically inseminated ewes there was a marked effect on the number of ewes from which spermatozoa were recovered of time of insemination and minor effects of time of flushing and of treatment of semen. Of the 36 ewes from which no spermatozoa were recovered 29 yielded eggs but none had been fertilized.

The estimated mean number of spermatozoa subsequently recovered from the fallopian tubes of 24 ewes 6 hr after cervical insemination at 0 and 24 hr after the detection of oestrus was 300 and 100 respectively. When the time of recovery was increased to 24 hr after both times of insemination the mean number of spermatozoa recovered was 4300 and 1200, representing a 14- and a 12-fold increase, respectively. The interaction between time of insemination and time of recovery was not significant. On the other hand, with uterine insemination, there was a highly significant ($P < 0\cdot001$) interaction between time of insemination and time of recovery. 17,100 and 28,900 spermatozoa were recovered 6 hr after insemination from ewes inseminated 0 and 24 hr, respectively, after detection of oestrus. However, the estimated mean number recovered 24 hr after insemination was 39,300 and 10,800 respectively.

IV. Discussion

It is apparent that the efficiency of transport of spermatozoa to the fallopian tubes was dependent upon the stage of oestrus at which ewes were inseminated. It is equally apparent that variations in fertilization were a direct reflection of the numbers of spermatozoa recovered from the fallopian tubes. In the ewe, the relationship between numbers of spermatozoa recovered from the fallopian tubes at about the time of ovulation—24 hr after the onset of oestrus—and fertilization has been well documented. Quinlivan and Robinson (1967) showed that the chances of fertilization occurring can be classed as slight, moderate, or high when less than 200, 200–6000, or more than 6000 spermatozoa were recovered from the tubes. Irrespective of time of insemination, uterine insemination resulted in mean spermatozoa numbers in excess of 10,000 and as could be expected fertilization rates were high. With cervical insemination comparable fertilization rates were only achieved in ewes which were inseminated at the onset of oestrus and a mean of 4300 spermatozoa were recovered from those ewes 24 hr after insemination. Cervical insemination 24 hr after the onset of oestrus depressed fertilization and the numbers of spermatozoa recovered at both 6 and 24 hr after insemination were so low that the chances of fertilization occurring could only be classed as moderate or slight. In fact no spermatozoa and no fertilized eggs were found in the flushings of more than half of the ewes cervically inseminated 24 hr after the onset of oestrus.

Increasing the time elapsing between cervical insemination at 24 hr and recovery of spermatozoa and eggs from 6 to 24 hr later did result in a build up in numbers of spermatozoa and some fertilized eggs were recovered, but the mean number of spermatozoa were still well below the number required for high fertilization rates. Even if these numbers increased still further with time, and this seems unlikely, it is very doubtful if any further increase in fertilization would occur. By 48 hr after the onset of oestrus the vast majority of eggs would have already lost their ability to become normally fertilized (Killeen and Moore 1970).

Mattner and Braden (1969) suggested that increased resistance of the cervical mucus of late oestrus to penetration by spermatozoa was primarily responsible for their poor transport late in oestrus. However, other sections of the tract may be involved. Early uterine insemination gave a twofold build up, between 6 and 24 hr, in numbers of tubal spermatozoa, whereas after late insemination there was a marked reduction in numbers between 6 and 24 hr. Either, spermatozoa were rapidly lost through expulsion or phagocytosis, or a barrier to movement of spermatozoa into the tubes became established in late oestrus.

At no time following uterine insemination were the numbers of spermatozoa in the tubes reduced to a level where fertilization was unlikely to occur. However, an excessive number $(3–4 \times 10^7)$ of live spermatozoa were injected into each uterine horn, whereas the maximum mean number of spermatozoa (live and dead) recovered by Quinlivan and Robinson (1969) from the uteri of ewes cervically inseminated with 50×10^7 spermatozoa was never greater than 88,000. The relatively high incidence of polyspermic eggs following uterine insemination was probably indicative of excessive numbers of spermatozoa in the vicinity of eggs at the time of fertilization.

Some fertilization can be achieved by surgical insemination as late as 54 hr after the onset of oestrus, but at 36 hr and beyond many of the fertilized eggs show gross nuclear abnormalities (Killeen and Moore 1970). The types of abnormalities encountered—polyspermy and multinucleate blastomeres—probably preclude normal full development. It is apparent that late cervical insemination or natural mating (if allowed by the ewe) is unlikely to provide sufficient tubal spermatozoa to achieve normal rates of fertilization. Thus, it appears that the ewe possesses an effective mechanism, operating through transportation of spermatozoa, that inhibits fertilization of aged eggs and the consequent reproductive wastage arising from the abnormalities associated with late fertilization.

Dilution with normal saline, and removal of seminal plasma by repeated washing did have minor effects upon the number of ewes from which spermatozoa were recovered, but neither had any effect upon fertilization. Clearly, as suggested by Dott (1964) seminal plasma plays little if any part in transport of spermatozoa, nor does the presence of seminal plasma in close proximity to recently ovulated eggs appear to have any marked effect on fertilization or early development of fertilized eggs. The effect of dilution and removal of seminal plasma on the numbers of spermatozoa recovered from the fallopian tubes was probably a simple reflection of effects of treatment on the viability of spermatozoa.

V. Acknowledgments

Grateful acknowledgment for technical assistance is made to Mr. A. J. Allison, Mr. A. D. Barnes, Mr. R. W. Connors, Mr. J. E. McRae, and Miss Narelle Flett.

Financial support was provided by the Australian Research Grants Committee and the Australian Wool Board. One of us (I.D.K.) was the recipient of a Wool Board Post-Graduate Fellowship.

VI. References

Chang, M. C. (1950).—The effect of seminal plasma on fertilized rabbit ova. *Proc. natn. Acad. Sci. U.S.A.* **36**, 188.

Dott, H. M. (1964).—Results of insemination with ram spermatozoa in different media. *J. Reprod. Fert.* **8**, 257.

HADEK, R. (1959).—Study of the sperm capacitation factor in the genital tract of the female rabbit. *Am. J. vet. Res.* **20**, 753.

HANCOCK, J. L. (1952).—The morphology of bull spermatozoa. *J. exp. Biol.* **29**, 445.

KILLEEN, I. D., and MOORE, N. W. (1970).—Fertilization and survival of fertilized eggs in the ewe following surgical insemination at various times after the onset of oestrus. *Aust. J. biol. Sci.* **23**, 1279.

MATTNER, P. E., and BRADEN, A. W. H. (1969).—Effect of time of insemination on the distribution of spermatozoa in the genital tract in ewes. *Aust. J. biol. Sci.* **22**, 1283.

QUINLIVAN, T. D., and ROBINSON, T. J. (1967).—The number of spermatozoa in the fallopian tubes of ewes at intervals after artificial insemination following withdrawal of SC-9880-impregnated intravaginal sponges. In "The Control of the Ovarian Cycle in the Sheep". (Ed. T. J. Robinson.) p. 177. (Sydney Univ. Press.)

QUINLIVAN, T. D., and ROBINSON, T. J. (1969).—Numbers of spermatozoa in the genital tract after artificial insemination of progestagen-treated ewes. *J. Reprod. Fert.* **19**, 73.

FERTILITY OF RAM SPERMATOZOA FROZEN BY THE PELLET METHOD

I. TRANSPORT AND VIABILITY OF SPERMATOZOA WITHIN THE GENITAL TRACT OF THE EWE

R. J. LIGHTFOOT AND S. SALAMON

INTRODUCTION

The infertility that normally accompanies insemination of ewes with frozen ram semen has been well documented (see reviews by Emmens, 1961; Emmens & Robinson, 1962; Sadleir, 1966), but until recently, little research has been conducted to investigate the reasons for the low fertility. Lopyrin & Loginova (1958) have reported that frozen ram spermatozoa penetrate more slowly to the cranial cervix than do those from fresh semen but the authors do not provide figures to substantiate this claim. Support for the theory of inadequate sperm transport is seen in the results of Loginova (1962), who was unable to recover any fertilized eggs from eight ewes following cervical insemination, whereas all three ewes examined after tubal insemination yielded fertilized eggs.

More recently, Salamon & Lightfoot (1967) found very low numbers of spermatozoa in the Fallopian tubes and a low fertilization rate following normal cervical insemination with pellet-frozen ram semen. When the cervix was by-passed by uterine insemination, however, fertilization rates of 88 and 93% were obtained. Similarly, Loginova & Zeltobrjuk (1968) have reported obtaining fertilization in two of sixteen and fifteen of seventeen ewes following cervical and tubal insemination, respectively. Working with ram semen frozen by the conventional slow freezing technique, Mattner, Entwistle & Martin (1969) studied the distribution of spermatozoa throughout the genital tract of ewes slaughtered either 4 or 24 hr after cervical insemination. They found comparatively few spermatozoa throughout the tract at 4 hr, while by 24 hr there were none in the uterus or Fallopian tubes and very few in the cervix. Both Loginova & Zeltobrjuk (1968) and Mattner *et al.* (1969) attributed the poor results with frozen semen to reduced viability of the spermatozoa *in vivo*.

The experiments reported here were conducted to examine more fully the transport and viability of frozen spermatozoa in the genital tract of the ewe, and in particular their early entry into the cervix.

MATERIALS AND METHODS

Experimental designs

Details of design and treatment comparisons for each of the four experiments are presented in Experimental Design and Results.

Sheep and management

Mature Merino ewes were used in all experiments, and were allocated at random to treatment groups on a within-draft basis. Oestrous ewes were detected with vasectomized rams fitted with Sire–sine harnesses and crayons (Radford, Watson & Wood, 1960). All vasectomized rams were previously tested by electro-ejaculation to ensure the absence of spermatozoa in the ejaculate.

In Exps 1, 2, 3 and 4b, the ewes were inseminated either during a natural cyclic oestrus or at the second oestrus after synchronization with intravaginal sponges (Syncro-Mate, Searle) impregnated with Cronolone (Robinson, 1965).

Experiment 4a was conducted in October, a season when most ewes at the location concerned are usually in anoestrus. The ewes were therefore injected intramuscularly (i.m.) with 1000 i.u. (reputed) pregnant mare serum gonadotrophin (G. D. Searle, Batch no. 2481) on the day of intravaginal-sponge withdrawal, and the ewes were inseminated at the resultant oestrus. The PMSG was subsequently assayed and found to be 2·2 times the stated potency, so, in fact, a dose of approximately 2200 i.u. was inadvertently administered.

Semen

Semen was collected from mature Merino rams by artificial vagina. For freezing, ejaculates of good initial motility were pooled and diluted 1 : 1 (Exp. 1) or 1 : 3 (Exps 2, 3 and 4) at 30° C with a diluent consisting of 166·5 mM-raffinose–102 mM-sodium citrate and 15% (v/v) egg yolk to which glycerol (6% v/v, Exp. 1; 5%, Exps 2 to 4) was added. The diluted semen was cooled to 5° C over a period of 1½ hr, then held at that temperature for an additional 3 to 6 hr before pellet-freezing (0·035 ml, Exps 1 and 4a; 0·35 ml, Exps 2, 3 and 4b) on dry ice. The pelleted semen was stored in liquid nitrogen for 2 to 12 weeks before use. Pellets were thawed in test tubes containing 88·4 mM-sodium citrate (2 : 1, pellets: thawing solution, v/v; in Exp. 1) or in 80·6 mM-sodium citrate–44·4 mM-glucose solution (1 : 3, Exps 2, 3 and 4) held in a water bath at 37° C. In the latter experiments, the thawed semen was centrifuged at 2500 rev/min for 15 min and the supernatant discarded to give the concentration of motile spermatozoa required for insemination.

For fresh semen, ejaculates of good initial motility were pooled then diluted to the required concentration of motile spermatozoa using either egg yolk–glucose–citrate (15%, v/v, 44·4 and 80·6 mM respectively) or, in Exp. 1, yolk–raffinose–citrate diluent. The concentration of both fresh and frozen semen was determined by haemocytometer, and the percentage motile spermatozoa by visual assessment (× 300) under a coverslip on a warm stage.

Insemination

Cervical inseminations (Exps 1, 2 and 3) were performed with the aid of a duck-billed speculum and headlight, the semen being deposited just inside or among the folds of the external cervical os. Particular care was taken in Exp. 3 to achieve a uniform 0·5 to 1·0 cm depth of insemination.

Uterine inseminations (Exp. 4) were performed following mid-ventral laparotomy under local anaesthesia. Semen was deposited into the cranial ipsilateral uterine horn by means of a sterile glass pipette with a fine glazed tip.

Oxytocin

The effect of oxytocin (Syntocinon, Sandoz) on the transport of spermatozoa and the fertilization of eggs was studied in Exp. 1. It was injected in physiological saline (1 ml, i.m.) into the hind leg at the time of insemination.

Recovery and counting of spermatozoa

Spermatozoa were recovered by flushing with physiological saline the appropriate regions of the genital tract of ewes under general anaesthesia (Exp. 1), local anaesthesia with sedation (Exp. 2), or following slaughter and removal of the genital tract (Exp. 3). The techniques used for recovery and counting of spermatozoa from the Fallopian tubes were as described by Quinlivan & Robinson (1967) for recovery and Mattner & Braden (1963) for counting, except that an eosin-fast green F.C.F. stain (Hackett & Macpherson, 1965) was used for staining the flushings before counting.

Ewes in Exp. 3 were killed 30 min after insemination by intra-cardiac injection of sodium pentobarbitone solution (5 ml, 600 mg/ml) and the genital tract was removed immediately after ligation of the utero-tubal and utero-cervical junctions. The Fallopian tubes and uteri were flushed with saline (1·5 and 20 ml respectively) and, after removal of the cervix, the vagina was flushed using a funnel to collect the washings. Extreme care was taken, with precautions similar to those adopted by Mattner & Braden (1963), to avoid contamination of flushings with spermatozoa from other regions. The flushings were frozen ($-15°$ C) and stored for subsequent counting of spermatozoa.

The cervices were separated from the remainder of the tract within 5 min of slaughter and were frozen rapidly by suspension in liquid nitrogen vapour, then stored at $-15°$ C. For counting spermatozoa, each cervix was cut transversely, using a new scalpel blade, into equal caudal, mid and cranial segments while still frozen. Each segment was then cut longitudinally into six slivers which were placed in a new vial containing 10 ml of physiological saline. When thawing was complete, the vials were allowed to stand for a further 30 min, and were shaken vigorously before samples were withdrawn for counting spermatozoa by the standard slide technique.

Egg recovery and fertilization
In Exps 1 and 4, eggs were recovered 48 to 60 hr after insemination (Nembutal anaesthesia, Exp. 1; local anaesthesia plus sedation, Exp. 4) and examined for cell cleavage. In Exp. 2, tubal flushings from ewes in which ovulation had occurred were examined before freezing and the numbers of spermatozoa on the zona pellucida of recovered eggs were recorded.

Statistical analyses
The statistical significance of treatment comparisons on the numbers of spermatozoa recovered from the genital tract (Exps 1a, 2 and 3) were determined by analysis of variance after transformation of the data according to the formula $\log_{10}$ (n+2). Arithmetic means are presented in the tables.

The effects of treatments on the proportions of eggs and ewes fertilized (Exps 1b and 4a) and on the distribution of fertilized eggs according to the number of spermatozoa on the zona pellucida (Exp. 4a) were in each case examined by analysis of χ^2 (Claringbold, 1961).

EXPERIMENTAL DESIGN AND RESULTS

EXPERIMENT 1

The effects of oxytocin and of insemination with fresh or frozen semen on the number of spermatozoa recovered from the Fallopian tubes and on fertilization were examined in Exp. 1. Exps 1a and 1b were conducted concurrently using the same flock of ewes and rams and the same insemination procedures.

Experiment 1a. Spermatozoa in the Fallopian tubes
The experiment was of factorial design: $2 \times 4 \times 3$; n $= 3$, N $= 72$.

(1) Semen type—fresh versus frozen
(2) Dose of oxytocin—0 versus 10 versus 20 i.u., i.m., at the time of insemination
(3) Time of flushing Fallopian tubes—3 versus 6 versus 12 versus 24 hr post-insemination.

Each ewe was inseminated once (cervical insemination) 10 to 25 hr after the onset of oestrus with 0·3 ml of semen containing 120×10^6 motile spermatozoa.

Table 1 shows the number of ewes from which spermatozoa were recovered and the mean numbers of spermatozoa/ewe according to treatments. Overall, spermatozoa were recovered from 72% of the ewes but the numbers recovered were generally low, none of the factors studied had a statistically significant effect, and there were no interactions.

TABLE 1

THE MEAN NUMBERS OF SPERMATOZOA RECOVERED FROM THE
FALLOPIAN TUBES AFTER CERVICAL INSEMINATION

Treatment	No. of ewes from which spermatozoa were recovered	Mean no. of spermatozoa /ewe
(1) *Type of semen* (n = 36)		
Fresh†	23	62
Frozen†	29	78
P	NS	NS
(2) *Time of recovery in hr after insemination* (n = 18)		
3	13	103
6	13	44
12	13	53
24	13	80
P	NS	NS
(3) *Dose (i.u.) of oxytocin* (n = 24)		
0	19	52
10	17	60
20	16	99
P	NS	NS

n = Number of ewes per comparison.
† Inseminate volume = 0·3 ml containing 120×10^6 motile spermatozoa $(0·4 \times 10^9/\text{ml})$.

Experiment 1b. Fertilization

The experiment was of factorial design: 2×3; n = 9 to 16 (number of ewes from which eggs were recovered), N = 70.

(1) Semen type—fresh versus frozen

(2) Dose of oxytocin—0 versus 10 versus 20 i.u., i.m. at the time of insemination.

The results are presented in Table 2. In all, eighty-eight ewes were inseminated and of these, seventy (80%) subsequently yielded a total of eighty-four eggs. There were no treatment effects upon the proportions either of eggs recovered or ewes from which eggs were recovered. Only twenty-two of the eighty-four eggs were fertilized (26·2%). Insemination with fresh semen resulted in seventeen fertilized eggs of thirty-eight eggs recovered, and with frozen semen in five of forty-six (44·7 versus 10·9%; $P < 0·001$). The administration of oxytocin significantly depressed the percentage of eggs fertilized and of ewes which yielded fertilized eggs ($P < 0·05$). Of the ewes that were not injected with oxytocin, fertilized eggs were recovered from 45·5% (five/eleven) and 31·3% (five/sixteen) following insemination with fresh and frozen spermatozoa respectively.

114

TABLE 2

THE EFFECTS OF TYPE OF SEMEN AND DOSE OF OXYTOCIN ON FERTILIZATION AFTER CERVICAL INSEMINATION

Treatment	No. of eggs			% of fertilized eggs	No. of ewes			% of ewes yielding fertilized eggs
	Ovulated	Recovered	Fertilized		Examined	Yielding eggs	Yielding fertilized eggs	
Dose of oxytocin (i.u.)								
0	43	34	13	38·2	35	27	10	37·0
10	34	26	7	26·9	28	22	5	22·7
20	34	24	2	8·3	25	21	2	9·5
P				<0·05				<0·05
Type of semen								
Fresh	48	38	17	44·7	35	30	12	40·0
Frozen	63	46	5	10·9	53	40	5	12·5
P				<0·001				<0·1
Overall	111	84	22	26·2	88	70	17	24·3

The effects of type of semen (fresh versus frozen) and of concentration of motile spermatozoa in frozen semen on the number of spermatozoa recoverable from the Fallopian tubes 24 hr after insemination were examined in Exp. 2.

There were three treatment groups, each of fourteen ewes; N = 42:

(1)—Frozen semen, 0.8×10^9 motile spermatozoa/ml
(2)—Frozen semen, 1.6×10^9 motile spermatozoa/ml
(3)—Fresh semen, 1.6×10^9 motile spermatozoa/ml

Each ewe was inseminated once (cervical insemination) with 0·1 ml of semen, 1 to 16 hr after the onset of oestrus.

The results are presented in Table 3. Spermatozoa were recovered from the Fallopian tubes of eighteen (64·3%) of the twenty-eight ewes examined 24 hr after insemination with frozen semen, whereas all fourteen ewes inseminated with fresh semen yielded spermatozoa ($P<0.05$). The mean numbers of spermatozoa recovered were 7741 and 575 for ewes inseminated with fresh and frozen semen respectively ($P<0.01$). There was no significant effect of concentration of motile spermatozoa in the frozen semen.

There was an apparent relationship between the percentage of eggs recovered with spermatozoa on the zona pellucida and the type of semen: frozen, 0.8×10^9, 22·2%; frozen, 1.6×10^9, 37·5%; fresh, 1.6×10^9, 62·5%.

EXPERIMENT 3

The effects of type of semen (fresh versus frozen) and of concentration of motile spermatozoa in frozen semen on the distribution of spermatozoa throughout the genital tract of ewes 30 min after insemination were examined in Exp. 3.

There were four treatment groups, each of eight animals; N = 32;

(1)—Frozen semen, 0.2×10^9 motile spermatozoa/ml
(2)—Frozen semen, 0.6×10^9 motile spermatozoa/ml
(3)—Frozen semen, 1.8×10^9 motile spermatozoa/ml
(4)—Fresh semen, 1.8×10^9 motile spermatozoa/ml

Each ewe was inseminated once (cervical insemination) with 0·1 ml of semen, 1 to 16 hr after the onset of oestrus.

Vagina. The mean numbers of spermatozoa found in the cranial vagina were 7·1, 32·1, 73·7 and 55·2 million for Treatments 1 to 4 and in each treatment represented approximately 20% of the total number inseminated (motile + non-motile). Some spermatozoa may have remained in the caudal vagina, which was not examined, but most of the loss was probably attributable to the drainage and/or expulsion of mucus with spermatozoa from the vagina between insemination and slaughter.

Cervix. The mean numbers for the caudal, mid and cranial regions of the cervix are shown in Table 4. The number increased as the concentration of spermatozoa in the frozen semen increased from 0·2 to 1.8×10^9 motile cells/ml ($P<0.001$), and insemination with fresh semen resulted in markedly higher numbers than with frozen semen ($P<0.01$), even with equivalent concentrations of motile spermatozoa.

117

TABLE 3

THE NUMBERS OF EGGS RECOVERED WITH SPERMATOZOA ON THE ZONA PELLUCIDA, THE NUMBERS OF EWES FROM WHICH SPERMATOZOA WERE RECOVERED FROM THE FALLOPIAN TUBES AND THE MEAN NUMBERS OF SPERMATOZOA RECOVERED/EWE 24 HR AFTER CERVICAL INSEMINATION

Treatment		No. of eggs		% of eggs with spermatozoa on the zona pellucida	Ewes from which spermatozoa were recovered		Mean no. of spermatozoa recovered
Type of semen	Concentration of motile spermatozoa ($\times 10^9$/ml)	Recovered	With spermatozoa on the zona pellucida		No.	%	
1. Frozen	0·8	9	2	22·2	10	71·4 } 64·3	345 } 575
2. Frozen	1·6	8	3	37·5	8	57·1	808
3. Fresh	1·6	8	5	62·5	14	100·0	7741
P				NS		<0·05	<0·01

Fourteen ewes/treatment.

There was a highly significant linear decline in the numbers of spermatozoa recovered from the caudal to the cranial region $(P \ll 0\cdot001)$ and there was no interaction between region and semen treatment, indicating that the rate of progression along the cervix, although variable, was similar in all treatments. However, the variability between ewes increased as spermatozoa were recovered from increasingly cranial regions of the cervix, as shown by the decreasing levels of significance of the regressions of the number of spermatozoa recovered on concentration of frozen semen (caudal, $P<0\cdot001$; mid, $P<0\cdot05$; cranial,

TABLE 4

THE EFFECTS OF TYPE OF SEMEN (FRESH VERSUS FROZEN)
AND OF CONCENTRATION OF MOTILE SPERMATOZOA IN FROZEN
SEMEN ON THE MEAN NUMBERS OF SPERMATOZOA RECOVERED
FROM THE CERVIX OF EWES 30 MIN AFTER INSEMINATION

Treatment		No. of spermatozoa ($\times 10^6$)			
		Region of cervix			
Type of semen	Conc. ($\times 10^9$ motile spermatozoa/ml)	Caudal	Mid	Cranial	Total cervix
1. Frozen	0·2	0·122	0·005	0·003	0·130
2. Frozen	0·6	0·448	0·039	0·002	0·489
3. Frozen	1·8	1·241	0·103	0·008	1·352
4. Fresh	1·8	7·031	0·537	0·042	7·610
Means		2·211	0·171	0·014	2·396

Summary of analysis of variance of the data in Table 4

Source of variation		d.f.	Mean square	Variance ratio
Semen treatment	(A)			
Fresh versus frozen semen		1		7·81**
Concentration of spermatozoa in frozen semen—linear		1		13·91***
—quadratic		1		0·15
Error 1 (Ewes within semen treatments)		28	3·39	
Cervical segment	(B)			
linear		1		98·99***
quadratic		1		1·49
A × B		6		1·05
Error 2—Residual		56	1·74	

$n = 8.$ ** $P<0\cdot01$;   *** $P<0\cdot001.$

$0\cdot05<P<0\cdot1$). The following regression $(P<0\cdot001)$ was calculated for total cervical spermatozoa:

$$y = 1\cdot75 + 1\cdot27x$$

$$\text{S.E.} = (\pm 0\cdot88)\ (\pm 0\cdot31)$$

where $y = \log_{10}$ number of spermatozoa in cervix,
$\quad x = \log_{10}$ concentration of motile spermatozoa ($\times 10^9$) in the inseminate (frozen semen).

118

TABLE 5

THE NUMBER OF EGGS RECOVERED AND THEIR CHARACTERISTICS FOLLOWING UTERINE INSEMINATION WITH FRESH OR FROZEN SPERMATOZOA

Treatment	No. of ewes inseminated	No. of eggs			% of eggs fertilized	No. of ewes		% of ewes yielding fertilized eggs	No. of fertilized eggs with spermatozoa on the zona pellucida		
		Ovulated	Recovered	Fertilized		Yielding eggs	Yielding fertilized eggs		0 to 1 sperm.	2 to 5 sperm.	>5 sperm.
Type of semen											
Fresh	30	94	40	31	77·5	19	16	84·2	1	10	20
Frozen	31	95	40	25	62·5	20	16	80·0	10	8	7
P					NS			NS		<0·01	
Time of uterine insemination*											
1 to 15 hr	29	81	35	26	74·3	19	14	73·7	7	9	10
12 to 26 hr	32	108	45	30	66·7	20	18	90·0	4	9	17
P					NS			NS		NS	

Note: The experiment was conducted in the spring months. Ewes were treated with progestagen-impregnated intravaginal sponges + PMSG and were inseminated at the resultant oestrus.

* Hours after onset of oestrus.

119

Uterus and Fallopian tubes. Spermatozoa were found in the uterine flushings of only four ewes of the thirty-two examined, two in Treatment 1 (6600 and 1,067,200 spermatozoa) and two in Treatment 4 (300 and 69,600). Spermatozoa were found in the tubal flushings of four ewes, only two of which yielded spermatozoa from the uterus. One of these was from Treatment 1 (3620) and one from Treatment 4 (20). The remaining two ewes were from Treatment 3 (1180 and 60).

EXPERIMENT 4

The experiment compared viability *in vivo* of frozen versus fresh spermatozoa as measured by the retention of fertilizing capacity following uterine insemination in (a) the spring months, using intravaginal progestagen treatment followed by PMSG and (b) in the autumn, using ewes in natural oestrus.

Experiment 4a

The experiment was of factorial design; 2×2; n = 9 or 10 (number of ewes from which eggs were recovered); N = 39:

(1) Type of semen—fresh versus frozen
(2) Time of uterine insemination—1 to 15 versus 12 to 26 hr after onset of oestrus.

All ewes were inseminated by the uterine method with 0·1 ml of semen containing 150×10^6 motile spermatozoa.

The results are presented in Table 5. Neither type of semen nor time of uterine insemination had a significant effect on the percentage of eggs recovered, eggs fertilized or ewes yielding fertilized eggs. Owing to the high dose of PMSG administered (see Materials and Methods), the time of ovulation was advanced considerably relative to the onset of oestrus. Thus, ovulation had already occurred in 20% of the ewes when inseminated 1 to 15 hr after the onset of oestrus and in 48% of ewes inseminated at 12 to 26 hr. There was no apparent effect of time of ovulation on fertilization. The use of fresh semen resulted in more eggs with large numbers of spermatozoa attached to the zona pellucida than did frozen semen ($P < 0.01$).

Experiment 4b

This was a simple comparison of the fertilizing capacity of fresh versus frozen spermatozoa when deposited into the uterus of ewes, in the normal breeding season, 1 to 6 hr after the onset of oestrus. Observations made during a concomitant experiment (Exp. 2) using the same flock of ewes indicated that ovulation occurred at the normal time, approximately 24 to 36 hr after the onset of oestrus. The uterine inseminations (0·1 ml containing 160×10^6 motile spermatozoa) were therefore performed approximately 18 to 35 hr before ovulation.

Ten ewes were inseminated with fresh and nine with frozen semen, and one egg was recovered from each of eight and six ewes, respectively. All eggs were fertilized and showed normal cell cleavage.

DISCUSSION

The importance of the cervix in the physiology of the transport of ovine spermatozoa has been well established (Quinlan, Maré & Roux, 1933; Starke, 1949; Dauzier & Wintenberger, 1952a; Dauzier, 1953; Mattner & Braden, 1963; Mattner, 1963, 1966). It constitutes the first barrier to the transport of spermatozoa through the genital tract, provides favourable environmental conditions for survival and acts as a reservoir from which spermatozoa continuously progress to the site of fertilization. The results reported here show the importance of two aspects involving the cervix in the failure of transport of spermatozoa following insemination with frozen semen. These are, first, the initial entry of spermatozoa into the cervix following insemination; and second, the viability of the spermatozoa *in vivo* which is associated with the maintenance of the cervical population.

Concerning the initial entry of spermatozoa into the cervix, the most significant observation was that the establishment of a cervical population was directly related to the concentration of motile spermatozoa in the inseminate (Exp. 3). It is possible that at very low concentrations the influence of dilution may be of more importance than the effects of freezing and thawing. Thus in Exp. 1, although insemination with frozen semen of low concentration resulted in the recovery of few spermatozoa from the Fallopian tubes, fresh semen, when diluted to the same low concentration of motile spermatozoa, produced equally poor results although the fertilization rate was higher. The results suggest that, for artificial insemination, the concentration of motile spermatozoa in the inseminate should be as high as possible, probably in the vicinity of $2 \cdot 0 \times 10^9$/ml. With ram semen frozen by the pellet method, this necessitates centrifugation immediately after thawing, as the use of very low dilution rates both before freezing and at thawing is associated with low revival rates and subsequent poor viability of the thawed spermatozoa (Lightfoot & Salamon, 1969a, b).

Following the establishment of the cervical population, the viability of frozen ram spermatozoa *in vivo* may be lower than that for fresh spermatozoa. Thus, Loginova & Zeltobrjuk (1968) reported that the viability of frozen spermatozoa in the ewe's genital tract after cervical insemination was only 12 hr, and fertilizing capacity was retained for no longer than 9 hr. More recently, Mattner *et al.* (1969) have attributed to reduced viability the low numbers of spermatozoa they found throughout the genital tract after insemination with frozen, compared with fresh, semen. Although their result may have been due in part to the lower concentration of motile spermatozoa in the frozen semen, it seems likely that the spermatozoa were less viable than those frozen rapidly by the pellet method and used in the experiments reported here. Hence, Mattner *et al.* (1969) found no spermatozoa in the Fallopian tubes 24 hr after insemination as compared with means of 92 and 808 spermatozoa from comparable treatments of Exps 1 and 2 reported here.

Further, the results of Exp. 4b show that a proportion of the pellet-frozen spermatozoa survived in the ewe's genital tract and retained the capacity to fertilize eggs for approximately 18 to 35 hr, compared with estimates of approximately 48 and 30 hr reported by Green (1947) and Dauzier & Wintenberger

(1952b) respectively for fresh spermatozoa. It should be noted, however, that Exp. 4b involved uterine insemination, by which means comparatively large numbers of spermatozoa can be established in the cervix (Lightfoot & Restall, unpublished). With normal cervical insemination and consequently fewer spermatozoa in the tract, the problem of low viability may assume added significance.

There are reports in several species, including swine (Milovanov & Sergeev, 1961; Jarosz, 1966) and cattle (Hays & VanDemark, 1952; Rowson, 1955; VanDemark & Hays, 1955), which indicate that the administration of oxytocin may increase the rate of transport of spermatozoa through the female genital tract. Published work with ewes is limited. Thibault & Wintenberger-Torres (1967) injected ewes with oxytocin (1·0 i.u., i.v.) after 30 min of unrestrained mating, but found no evidence for an increased rate of transport. However, Lang & Oh (1968) claimed that whereas injections of 0·1 i.u. had no effect, 1·0 i.u. depressed the numbers of spermatozoa recovered from the Fallopian tubes 16 hr after mating. The high doses (10 and 20 i.u.) used in the present study did not affect the number of spermatozoa recovered from the Fallopian tubes, but such treatment significantly depressed fertility—an effect which has been confirmed in subsequent experiments (Salamon & Lightfoot, 1970).

In conclusion, it appears that the low fertilization rate obtained following insemination with pellet-frozen ram semen is due to the failure in the normal pattern of transport and consequently low numbers of motile spermatozoa in the genital tract of the ewe. Embryonic mortality following cervical insemination with pellet-frozen ram semen is of a similar magnitude to that found with fresh semen(Lightfoot & Salamon, 1970). Therefore, procedures that effectively aid the initial establishment of the cervical population of spermatozoa, such as increasing the concentration of motile spermatozoa in the thawed semen and double insemination, result in improved lambing performance (Salamon & Lightfoot, 1970).

ACKNOWLEDGMENTS

The authors are indebted to Mr J. L. Hodgkinson and Sons, Vale View, Yass, N.S.W., for their generous provision of sheep and facilities in Experiment 4, to Mr B. M. Bindon for conducting PMSG assays, and to Sandoz Australia Pty Ltd for donations of oxytocin.

We wish to thank Professor T. J. Robinson for his comments on the manuscript. The research was aided by grants from the Australian Wool Board and the Australian Research Grants Committee.

REFERENCES

CLARINGBOLD, P. J. (1961) The use of orthogonal polynomials in the partition of chi-square. *Aust. J. Statistics*, **3**, 48.

DAUZIER, L. (1953) Recherches sur les facteurs de la remontée des spermatozoïdes dans les voies génitales femelles. Étude chez la brebis (col de l'utérus). *C. r. Séanc. Soc. Biol.* **147**, 1556.

DAUZIER, L. & WINTENBERGER, S. (1952a) La vitesse de remontée des spermatozoïdes dans le tractus génital de la brebis. *Annls Zootech.* **1**, 13.

DAUZIER, L. & WINTENBERGER, S. (1952b) Recherches sur la fécondation chez les mammifères: Durée du pouvoir fécondant des spermatozoïdes de bélier dans le tractus génital de la brebis et durée de la période de fécondité de l'œuf après 'olvulation. *C. r. Séanc. Soc. Biol.* **146**, 660.

B

EMMENS, C. W. (1961) *Dilution, transport and storage of ram semen.* In: Artificial Breeding of Sheep in Australia, p. 118. Proc. Conf. School of Wool Technology, University of N.S.W., Australia.

EMMENS, C. W. & ROBINSON, T. J. (1962) Artificial insemination in the sheep. In: The Semen of Animals and Artificial Insemination. *Tech. Commun. Commonw. Bur. Anim. Breed. Genet.* **15**, 205.

GREEN, W. W. (1947) Duration of sperm fertility in the ewe. *Am. J. vet. Res.* **8**, 299.

HACKETT, A. J. & MACPHERSON, J. W. (1965) Some staining procedures for spermatozoa. A review. *Can. vet. J.* **6**, 55.

HAYS, R. L. & VANDEMARK, N. L. (1952) The effect of hormones on uterine motility and sperm transport in the perfused genital tract of the cow. *J. Dairy Sci.* **35**, 499.

JAROSZ, S. (1966) The effect of hypophysin introduced into the uterus on sperm transport in the uterus and oviducts of the sow. *Roczn. Nauk. roln.* Ser. B, **88**, 19. (*Anim. Breed. Abstr.* **36**, No. 604).

LANG, D. R. & OH, K. Y. (1968) Distribution of spermatozoa in the reproductive tract of the Romney ewe. *Proc. N.Z. Soc. Anim. Prod.* **28**, 120.

LIGHTFOOT, R. J. SALAMON, S. (1969a) Freezing ram spermatozoa by the pellet method. II. The effects of method of dilution, dilution rate, glycerol concentration and duration of storage at 5°C prior to freezing on survival of spermatozoa. *Aust. J. biol. Sci.* **22**, 1547.

LIGHTFOOT, R. J. & SALAMON, S. (1969b) Freezing ram spermatozoa by the pellet method. III. The effects of pellet volume, composition of the thawing solution and reconcentration of the thawed semen on survival of spermatozoa. *Aust. J. biol. Sci.* **22**, 1561.

LIGHTFOOT, R. J. & SALAMON, S. (1970) Fertility of ram spermatozoa frozen by the pellet method. II. The effects of method of insemination on fertilization and embryonic mortality. *J. Reprod. Fert.* **22**, 399.

LOGINOVA, N. V. (1962) Causes of low fertility in ewes inseminated with frozen semen. *Ovtsevodstvo,* **8**(8), 20.

LOGINOVA, N. V. & ZELTOBRJUK, N. A. (1968) Test of different methods of freezing semen. *Ovtsevodstvo,* **14**(9), 22.

LOPYRIN, A. I. & LOGINOVA, N. V. (1958) Method of freezing ram semen. *Ovtsevodstvo,* **4**(8), 31.

MATTNER, P. E. (1963) Spermatozoa in the genital tract of the ewe. II. Distribution after coitus. *Aust. J. biol. Sci.* **16**, 688.

MATTNER, P. E. (1966) Formation and retention of the spermatozoan reservoir in the cervix of the ruminant. *Nature, Lond.* **212**, 1479.

MATTNER, P. E. & BRADEN, A. W. H. (1963) Spermatozoa in the genital tract of the ewe. I. Rapidity of transport. *Aust. J. biol. Sci.* **16**, 473.

MATTNER, P. E. ENTWISTLE, K. W. & MARTIN, I. C. A. (1969) Passage, survival and fertility of deep-frozen ram semen in the genital tract of the ewe. *Aust. J. biol. Sci.* **22**, 181.

MILOVANOV, V. K. & SERGEEV, N. I. (1961) The simultaneous use of oxytocin—a new method of increasing the effectiveness of artificial insemination of pigs. *Zhivotnovodstvo, Mosk.* **23**(11), 70.

QUINLAN, J., MARÉ, G. S. & ROUX, L. L. (1933) A study of the duration of motility of spermatozoa in the different divisions of the reproductive tract of the Merino sheep. *Onderstepoort J. vet. Res.* **1**, 135.

QUINLIVAN, T. D. & ROBINSON, T. J. (1967) *The number of spermatozoa in the fallopian tubes of ewes at intervals after artificial insemination following withdrawal of SC-9880-impregnated intravaginal sponges.* In: The Control of the Ovarian Cycle in the Sheep, p. 177. Ed. T. J. Robinson. Sydney University Press.

RADFORD, H. M., WATSON, R. H. & WOOD, G. F. (1960) A crayon and associated harness for the detection of mating under field conditions. *Aust. vet. J.* **36**, 57.

ROBINSON, T. J. (1965) Use of progestagen-impregnated sponges inserted intravaginally or subcutaneously for the control of the oestrous cycle in the sheep. *Nature, Lond.* **206**, 39.

ROWSON, L. E. A. (1955) The movement of radio opaque material in the bovine uterine tract. *Br. vet. J.* **111**, 334.

SADLEIR, R. M. F. S. (1966) The preservation of mammalian spermatozoa by freezing. *Lab. Pract.* **15**, 413.

SALAMON, S. & LIGHTFOOT, R. J. (1967) Fertilisation and embryonic loss in sheep after insemination with deep frozen semen. *Nature, Lond.* **216**, 194.

SALAMON, S. & LIGHTFOOT, R. J. (1970) Fertility of ram spermatozoa frozen by the pellet method. III. The effects of insemination technique, oxytocin and relaxin on lambing. *J. Reprod. Fert.* **22**, 409.

STARKE, N. C. (1949) The sperm picture of rams of different breeds as an indication of their fertility. II. The rate of sperm travel in the genital tract of the ewe. *Onderstepoort J. vet. Res.* **22**, 415.

THIBAULT, C. & WINTENBERGER-TORRES, S. (1967) Oxytocin and sperm transport in the ewe. *Int. J. Fert.* **12**, 410.

VANDEMARK, N. L. & HAYS, R. L. (1955) Sperm transport in the perfused genital tract of the cow. *Am. J. Physiol.* **183**, 510.

123

FERTILITY OF RAM SPERMATOZOA FROZEN BY THE PELLET METHOD

II. THE EFFECTS OF METHOD OF INSEMINATION ON FERTILIZATION AND EMBRYONIC MORTALITY

R. J. LIGHTFOOT AND S. SALAMON

INTRODUCTION

Lightfoot & Salamon (1970) have shown that the infertility following insemination with pellet-frozen ram semen was associated with an impaired pattern
of transport of spermatozoa in the ewe's genital tract. This was due to failure
to establish and maintain an adequate cervical population of spermatozoa, a
problem which was partly overcome by using inseminates with a high concentration of motile spermatozoa. The results suggested that concentration of the
thawèd semen before insemination should result in improved fertility.

In an earlier study, Salamon & Lightfoot (1967) obtained high fertilization
rates (88% and 93%) when the cervix was by-passed, by depositing frozen
semen directly into the uterus, but subsequent survival of the zygotes was poor.
Of sixty-eight ewes inseminated and retained for lambing, only twenty-three
(34%) had not returned to service 22 days later, and only seventeen (25%)
subsequently lambed.

In view of this evidence, the experiment reported here was designed to
examine ewe fertility:

124

(i) when the cervical population of spermatozoa was increased by using inseminates containing a high concentration of motile spermatozoa;

(ii) when the cervical barrier to sperm transport was by-passed by surgical insemination into the uterus.

Both fertilization and lambing were studied to determine whether, following insemination with frozen semen, excessive embryonic mortality further contributed to reduced ewe fertility, in addition to failure of fertilization.

MATERIALS AND METHODS

Experimental design

The experiment was of factorial design, $3 \times 2 \times 2$, n = 22 to 40, N = 362, as shown below.

(1) Method of insemination—cervical versus cervical traction versus uterine
(2) Type of semen—fresh versus frozen
(3) Stage of pregnancy—fertilization versus lambing

Sheep and management

Mature Merino ewes were allocated at random to treatments on a within draft basis. The methods adopted for testing vasectomized rams before joining and identifying ewes in oestrus were as described previously (Lightfoot & Salamon, 1970). Oestrous ewes were drafted from the flock at 07.00 hours daily. Ewes allocated to the cervical and cervical traction methods of insemination were inseminated twice, first within 3 hr of drafting (approximately 1 to 27 hr after onset of oestrus), and again 12 hr later. Ewes inseminated by the uterine method received one insemination 9 to 39 hr after the onset of oestrus. All inseminations were performed with 0·1 ml of semen containing 160×10^6 motile spermatozoa. Cervical (external os) and uterine inseminations were as described earlier (Lightfoot & Salamon, 1970). For cervical traction inseminations, a cervical papilla was grasped with a long pair of forceps and the cervical os withdrawn to a position just cranial of the vaginal entrance.

Semen

For freezing, semen was collected by artificial vagina and diluted (1 : 3, semen : diluent, v/v) at 30° C with a diluent consisting of 166·5 mм-raffinose, 102 mм-sodium citrate, 15% (v/v) egg yolk to which was added 5% (v/v) glycerol. The diluted semen was cooled over 1½ hr to 5° C, held at that temperature for 3 hr, then frozen as pellets (0·035 ml) on dry ice and stored in liquid nitrogen for 2 to 12 weeks before use. The pellets were thawed (1 : 3, pellets : thawing solution, v/v) in 44·4 mм-glucose–80·6 mм-sodium citrate at 37° C. The thawed semen was centrifuged at 2500 rev/min for 15 min and the supernatant discarded to achieve a concentration of $1·6 \times 10^9$ motile spermatozoa/ml for insemination.

The fresh semen was collected from two rams and the concentration of spermatozoa was determined by haemocytometer after pooling the ejaculates. The semen was then diluted two- to three-fold with egg yolk–glucose–citrate diluent (15% by vol, 44·4 mм and 80·6 mм respectively) to a concentration of $1·6 \times 10^9$ motile spermatozoa/ml for insemination.

Fertilization

Eggs were recovered 48 to 60 hr after insemination following mid-ventral laparotomy under local anaesthesia. The eggs were examined for cell cleavage, presence of polar bodies and number of spermatozoa on the zona pellucida.

Lambing

Vasectomized rams were joined with ewes in the lambing treatments to obtain individual non-return records. The ewes were side-numbered 2 weeks before the commencement of lambing and individual ewe records obtained by drift-lambing (Tribe & Coles, 1966) with twice daily inspections.

Statistical analyses

The statistical significance of all treatment comparisons was determined by analysis of χ^2 (Claringbold, 1961).

RESULTS

Data for ovulation, egg recovery and egg fertilization are presented in Table 1. A slightly lower proportion of eggs was recovered following uterine insemination than after insemination by the cervical and cervical traction methods (73·0%, 85·0% and 82·3%, respectively; surgical versus non-surgical insemination, $\chi_1^2 = 2·91$; $0·05 < P < 0·1$).

TABLE 1

OVULATION, EGG RECOVERY AND EGG FERTILIZATION AFTER CERVICAL, CERVICAL TRACTION AND UTERINE INSEMINATION WITH FRESH AND FROZEN RAM SPERMATOZOA

Treatment		No. of ewes inseminated for estimates of fertilization	No. of eggs			% of eggs	
Method of insemination	Type of semen		Ovulated	Recovered	Fertilized	Recovered	Fertilized
Cervical	Fresh	23	31	27	19	87·1	70·4
	Frozen	24	29	24	11	82·8	45·8
Cervical traction	Fresh	30	33	25	17	75·8	68·0
	Frozen	22	29	26	11	89·7	42·3
Uterine	Fresh	26	32	23	20	71·9	87·0
	Frozen	28	31	23	21	74·2	91·3
Overall		153	185	148	99	80·0	66·9

The use of frozen semen, as compared with fresh, resulted in a lower proportion of eggs fertilized following both cervical (45·8% versus 70·4%) and cervical traction (42·3% versus 68·0%) insemination. Frozen and fresh semen were of equal fertility, (91·3% versus 87·0%), however, when inseminated into the uterus (type of semen × method of insemination, non-surgical versus surgical: $\chi_1^2 = 3·49$; $0·05 < P < 0·1$).

The effects of method of insemination, type of semen and stage of pregnancy on ewe fertility are shown in Table 2 and the relevant analysis of χ^2 in Table 3. Two main points emerge from these comparisons.

126

TABLE 2

THE EFFECTS OF METHOD OF INSEMINATION AND TYPE OF SEMEN ON FERTILIZATION, LAMBING AND ESTIMATED EMBRYONIC MORTALITY

Treatment		Stage of pregnancy						Estimated embryonic mortality (%)*
		Fertilization			Lambing			
Method of insemination	Type of semen	No. of ewes		% of ewes yielding fertilized eggs	No. of ewes		% of ewes lambing	
		Yielding eggs	Yielding fertilized eggs		Inseminated	Lambing		
Cervical	Fresh	21	16	76·2	35	24	68·6	10·0
	Frozen	19	11	57·9	40	20	50·0	13·6
Cervical traction	Fresh	24	16	66·7	36	27	75·0	—
	Frozen	21	9	42·9	37	11	29·7	30·8
Uterine	Fresh	19	17	89·5	31	17	54·8	38·8
	Frozen	21	19	90·5	30	12	40·0	55·8
Main effects								
Cervical	Fresh	40	27	67·5	75	44	58·7	13·0
	Frozen	45	25	55·6	73	38	52·1	6·3
Cervical traction		40	36	90·0	61	29	47·5	47·2
Uterine	Fresh	64	49	76·6	102	68	66·7	12·9
	Frozen	61	39	63·9	107	43	40·2	37·1
Overall		125	88	70·4	209	111	53·1	24·6

* 100 (% Fertilization minus % Lambing/% Fertilization) %.

(i) Frozen semen was of lower fertility than fresh semen (63·9% fertilization, 40·2% lambing, mean = 48·8% versus 76·6%, 66·7%, mean = 70·5%; $P < 0\cdot001$).

(ii) There was a significant interaction between stage of pregnancy and

TABLE 3

ANALYSIS OF χ^2 OF DATA IN TABLE 2

Effect		d.f.	χ^2
Method of insemination (M)			
Within non-surgical†		1	1·69
Non-surgical versus surgical‡		1	1·37
Semen type (S)		1	16·29***
Stage of pregnancy (P)			
Fertilization versus lambing		1	9·71**
M × S			
Within non-surgical × S		1	1·98
Non-surgical versus surgical × S		1	3·16
M × P			
Within non-surgical × P		1	0·14
Non-surgical versus surgical × P		1	9·90**
S × P		1	1·46
M × S × P		2	0·61

** $P < 0\cdot01$;   *** $P < 0\cdot001$.
† Cervical versus cervical traction.
‡ Cervical and cervical traction versus uterine.

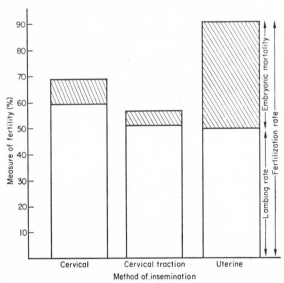

TEXT-FIG. 1. The effect of method of insemination on the incidence of embryonic mortality. (Method of insemination, non-surgical versus surgical × stage of pregnancy, $P < 0\cdot01$). Data are the means of fresh and frozen semen treatments.

method of insemination ($P < 0.01$). Thus, following insemination by the cervical and cervical traction (non-surgical) methods, lambing rates were only slightly lower than fertilization rates (13·0% and 6·3% estimated embryonic mortality respectively), but following uterine (surgical) insemination, lambing rates were much lower than fertilization rates (47·2% estimated embryonic mortality). This relationship is shown in Text-fig. 1. Results for both fresh and frozen semen treatments were similar in this respect.

The overall estimates of embryonic mortality following insemination with fresh and frozen semen were 12·9% and 37·1% respectively. This difference, examined statistically by the interaction between type of semen and stage of pregnancy, however, was not significant ($\chi_1^2 = 1.46$; $0.2 < P < 0.3$).

Fertilized eggs were classified according to the number of spermatozoa counted on the zona pellucida immediately after recovery (Table 4). Insemination with fresh, as compared with frozen, semen resulted in a greater proportion of eggs to which numerous spermatozoa were attached ($P < 0.01$). Both

TABLE 4

CLASSIFICATION OF FERTILIZED EGGS ACCORDING TO THE NUMBER OF
SPERMATOZOA ON THE ZONA PELLUCIDA

Treatment	No. of eggs with spermatozoa on the zona pellucida				Mean no. of spermatozoa on zona pellucida
	0 sperm.	1 to 5 sperm.	6 to 20 sperm.	> 20 sperm.	
Type of semen					
Fresh	7	18	13	18	19·4
Frozen	5	24	12	2	6·0
P			< 0·01		
Method of insemination					
Cervical	8	12	7	3	8·1
Cervical traction	2	13	5	8	17·0
Uterine	2	17	13	9	15·3
P			$0.05 < P < 0.1$		

the uterine and cervical traction insemination procedures tended to yield a higher proportion of fertilized eggs with large numbers of spermatozoa on the zona pellucida ($0.05 < P < 0.10$). When both these methods were tested collectively against cervical insemination, the difference was statistically significant ($P < 0.05$).

Of the ewes that failed to lamb, approximately 80% returned to service (vasectomized rams) within 24 days of insemination and this proportion was similar in all treatments.

There were no differences between treatments in the number of blastomeres in fertilized eggs.

Of the fifty-four ewes subjected to laparotomy and uterine insemination, and in which fertilization was examined, twenty-four were inseminated before and thirty after ovulation. Of the forty-six eggs subsequently recovered, only four were unfertilized (two fresh and two frozen semen), all from ewes inseminated after ovulation. Table 5 shows no effect on lambing performance, following

TABLE 5

LAMBING DATA IN RELATION TO WHETHER UTERINE INSEMINATION WAS PERFORMED BEFORE OR AFTER OVULATION

	No. of ewes								
	Time of uterine insemination						Overall		
	Before ovulation			After ovulation					
Main effect	Inseminated	Lambed	%	Inseminated	Lambed	%	Inseminated	Lambed	%
Type of semen									
Fresh	16	8	50·0	15	9	60·0	31	17	54·8
Frozen	20	8	40·0	10	4	40·0	30	12	40·0
Overall	36	16	44·4	25	13	52·0	61	29	47·5

130

the use of either fresh or frozen semen, attributable to time of uterine insemination relative to ovulation.

DISCUSSION

The relatively low fertilization rates that normally accompany insemination with deep-frozen ram semen can be markedly increased by depositing the spermatozoa directly into the uterus. Eggs fertilized following insemination by this technique are characterized by numerous spermatozoa on the zona pellucida, indicating that uterine insemination improves fertilization by increasing the number of spermatozoa that reach the Fallopian tubes.

Despite the achievement of high fertilization rates with frozen spermatozoa by uterine insemination, lambing results were poor, due presumably to the occurrence of excessive embryonic mortality. This phenomenon occurred following uterine inseminations with either fresh or frozen spermatozoa in contrast to the occurrence of normal levels of embryonic mortality (Quinlivan, Martin, Taylor & Cairney, 1966a, b; Mattner & Braden, 1967) following normal cervical insemination. High embryonic losses following uterine insemination with both fresh and frozen spermatozoa is suggested by the data of Mattner Entwistle & Martin (1969) but few animals were involved and there were no normal insemination controls.

The physiological mechanisms by which surgical insemination in the sheep precipitates excessive embryonic losses are not clear. The uteri showed no response on macroscopic examination 2 days after insemination but most ewes returned to service at the normal time. From the results of Moor & Rowson (1966), this indicates that the zygotes died before Day 12. It is possible that the surgical interference brought about a response of the genital tract leading to reduced survival of otherwise normal zygotes, or to a high incidence of abnormal zygotes due to anomalous fertilization.

There are several Soviet reports concerned with excessive embryonic mortality in the ewe after surgical insemination with fresh semen (Lopyrin & Loginova, 1957; Lopyrin, Loginova & Zeltobrjuk, 1965; Lopyrin & Rak, 1965; Lopyrin & Manujlov, 1966, 1967). It has been claimed that both the semen diluent and dilution rate may affect the extent of losses found, but there were too few animals involved in most treatment comparisons to permit the drawing of valid conclusions.

The cervical traction method of insemination offered no advantage over normal cervical insemination, in contrast to earlier promising results (Salamon & Lightfoot, 1967) and the findings of Ten En Bon (1965).

There have been few reports concerned with the comparative levels of embryonic mortality following non-surgical inseminations with fresh and frozen spermatozoa. Shaffner (1942) reported that twelve of forty-eight eggs produced by hens after insemination with frozen spermatozoa were fertile, but embryonic development did not proceed for more than 10 to 15 hr. More recently, Wales & O'Shea (1968) and O'Shea & Wales (1969) have achieved limited fertility with deep-frozen spermatozoa in the rabbit, but they found no evidence that embryonic mortality was increased. Excessive embryonic mortality is unlikely to occur following insemination with pellet-frozen bull spermatozoa, as fertility is usually similar to that obtained with chilled semen (e.g. Leipnitz, 1965; Milk Marketing Board, 1965/66; Meding, 1966). There appear to be no studies on early embryonic mortality, but comparisons of early versus late non-return rates for cows inseminated with bull spermatozoa frozen in ampoules (Salisbury, 1963, 1967) have indicated pre-natal losses of an order similar to that reported for semen after short-term liquid storage (Salisbury & Flerchinger, 1967).

In the present study, embryonic mortality in ewes inseminated with frozen spermatozoa was not significantly higher than that observed with fresh semen. This is in agreement with a recent report by Volkov (1968) who found fertilization and lambing rates of 11·9% and 15·8% respectively, following inseminations with ram semen frozen by the pellet method in a lactose–yolk diluent. Normal cervical inseminations with concentrated frozen spermatozoa in the present experiment resulted in fertilization and lambing rates of 57·9% and 50·0% respectively. Thus, losses due to embryonic mortality were of lesser importance than failure of fertilization due to impaired transport of spermatozoa.

ACKNOWLEDGMENTS

We thank the Western Australian Department of Agriculture, and in particular Mr H. G. Neil, for providing sheep and facilities; Mr K. P. Croker and Mr R. O'Farrell for their assistance; and Professor T. J. Robinson for interest and discussion. The research was aided by grants from the Australian Wool Board and the Australian Research Grants Committee.

REFERENCES

CLARINGBOLD, P. J. (1961) The use of orthogonal polynomials in the partition of chi-square. *Aust. J. Statistics*, **3**, 48.

LEIPNITZ, CHR. (1965) Routinebesamung mit Tiefkühlsperma, dass in Pillenform gefroren wurde. *Dt. tierärztl. Wschr.* **72**, 469.

LIGHTFOOT, R. J. & SALAMON, S. (1970) Fertility of ram spermatozoa frozen by the pellet method. I. Transport and viability of spermatozoa within the genital tract of the ewe. *J. Reprod. Fert.* **22**, 385.

LOPYRIN, A. I. & LOGINOVA, N. V. (1957) Experimental verification of the effect of sperm quality on the vitality of the progeny of sheep. *Dokl. vses. Akad. sel'.-khoz. Nauk.* **22**(s), 40.

LOPYRIN, A. I., LOGINOVA, N. V. & ZELTOBRJUK, N. A. (1965) Causes of high embryonic mortality after intra-tubal insemination in sheep. *Ovtsevodstvo*, **11**(8), 3.

LOPYRIN, A. I. & MANUJLOV, I. M. (1966) Biological control of the diluents for ram semen. *Ovtsevodstvo*, **12**(9), 21.

LOPYRIN, A. I. & MANUJLOV, I. M. (1967) Insemination of ewes with small doses of semen. *Ovtsevodstvo*, **13**(9), 34.

LOPYRIN, A. I. & RAK, L. P. (1965) Embryonic viability and the quality of the lambs in relation to the age of the gametes. *Vest. sel. '-khoz. Nauki, Mosk.* **10**, 50.

MATTNER, P. E. & BRADEN, A. W. H. (1967) Studies in flock mating of sheep. II. Fertilization and prenatal mortality. *Aust. J. exp. Agric. Anim. Husb.* **7**, 110.

MATTNER, P. E., ENTWISTLE, K. W. & MARTIN, I. C. A. (1969) Passage, survival and fertility of deep-frozen ram semen in the genital tract of the ewe. *Aust. J. biol. Sci.* **22**, 181.

MEDING, J. H. (1966) *The use of deep-frozen pelleted semen.* In: Annual Report, The Royal Veterinary and Agricultural College, Sterility Research Institute, Copenhagen, p. 179.

MILK MARKETING BOARD (1965/66) Report of the breeding and production organisation. Thames Ditton, Surrey. No. **16**, p. 118.

MOOR, R. M. & ROWSON, L. E. A. (1966) The corpus luteum of the sheep: effect of the removal of embryos on luteal function. *J. Endocr.* **34**, 497.

O'SHEA, T. & WALES, R. G. (1969) Further studies of the deep freezing of rabbit spermatozoa in reconstituted skim milk powder. *Aust. J. biol. Sci.* **22,** 709.

QUINLIVAN, T. D., MARTIN, C. A., TAYLOR, W. B. & CAIRNEY, I. M. (1966a) Estimates of pre- and perinatal mortality in the New Zealand Romney Marsh ewe. I. Pre- and perinatal mortality in those ewes that conceived to one service. *J. Reprod. Fert.* **11,** 379.

QUINLIVAN, T. D., MARTIN, C. A., TAYLOR, W. B. & CAIRNEY, I. M. (1966b) Estimates of pre- and perinatal mortality in the New Zealand Romney Marsh ewe. II. Pre- and perinatal loss in those ewes that conceived to second service and were mated a third time. *J. Reprod. Fert.* **11,** 391.

SALAMON, S. & LIGHTFOOT, R. J. (1967) Fertilization and embryonic loss in sheep after insemination with deep frozen semen. *Nature, Lond.* **216,** 194.

SALISBURY, G. W. (1963) Effect of ageing at −79°C on fertility of bovine semen. *J. Dairy Sci.* **46,** 637.

SALISBURY, G. W. (1967) Aging phenomena in spermatozoa. III. Effect of season and storage at −79 to −88°C on fertility and prenatal losses. *J. Dairy Sci.* **50,** 1683.

SALISBURY, G. W. & FLERCHINGER, F. H. (1967) Aging phenomena in spermatozoa. I. Fertility and prenatal losses with use of liquid semen. *J. Dairy Sci.* **50,** 1675.

SHAFFNER, C. S. (1942) Longevity of fowl spermatozoa in frozen condition. *Science, N.Y.* **96,** 33.

TEN EN BON (1965) Physiological and biochemical characters of semen should be considered by insemination with frozen semen. *Ovtsevodstvo,* **11**(8), 11.

TRIBE, D. E. & COLES, G. J. R. (1966) *Management of lambing ewes.* In: Prime Lamb Production, p. 78. F. W. Cheshire, Melbourne.

VOLKOV, A. S. (1968) Conception in ewes inseminated with deep frozen semen. *Sb. nauch. Rab. vses. Ord. Trud. krasn. Znam. nauchno-issled. Inst. Zhivot.,* No. **10,** 74. (*Anim. Breed. Abstr.* **37,** No. 593).

WALES, R. G. & O'SHEA, T. (1968) The deep freezing of rabbit spermatozoa. *Aust. J. biol. Sci.* **21,** 831.

FERTILITY OF RAM SPERMATOZOA FROZEN BY THE PELLET METHOD

III. THE EFFECTS OF INSEMINATION TECHNIQUE, OXYTOCIN AND RELAXIN ON LAMBING

S. SALAMON AND R. J. LIGHTFOOT

INTRODUCTION

Lambing results following cervical insemination with ram spermatozoa frozen rapidly by the pellet method are generally low. Salamon (1967) obtained only 6% ewes lambing, Platov (1968) 2% to 24%, Loginova & Zeltobrjuk (1968) 27%, Fraser (1968) 31% and Volkov (1968) 16%.

The causes of reproductive failure following insemination with ram spermatozoa frozen by the pellet method were investigated by Lightfoot & Salamon (1970a) who found that the transport of spermatozoa through the ewe's genital tract was primarily affected. The results demonstrated a failure of the establishment and maintenance of the cervical population of spermatozoa which could be partly overcome by use of inseminates with a high concentration of motile spermatozoa. The work also showed (Lightfoot & Salamon, 1970b) that embryonic mortality following cervical insemination with pellet frozen spermatozoa was of similar magnitude to that obtained with fresh semen, confirming that most reproductive wastage occurred before fertilization. Using double cervical insemination with thawed semen of high concentration, a lambing rate of 50% was obtained.

In view of these results, the experiments presented here were conducted to examine procedures that might enhance the transport of spermatozoa through the ewe's genital tract and therefore increase fertilization and lambing rates. The hormones, oxytocin and relaxin were also included in the study as there was reason to suspect that suitable therapy might influence sperm transport.

MATERIALS AND METHODS

Experimental designs

Details of design and treatment comparisons for each of the five experiments are presented in Experimental Designs and Results.

Sheep and management

Mature Merino ewes were used in all experiments and were allocated at random to treatments on a 'within draft' basis. The methods adopted for testing vasectomized rams before using them to identify ewes in oestrus, were as described previously (Lightfoot & Salamon, 1970a).

Semen

Semen was collected from mature Merino rams by artificial vagina. Ejaculates of good initial motility were pooled and diluted 1 : 1 (Exp. 1) or 1 : 3 (Exps 2 to 5) at 30° C with a diluent consisting of 166·5 mM-raffinose, 102 mM-sodium citrate, 15% v/v egg yolk to which glycerol (6% v/v, Exp. 1; 5%, Exps 2 to 5) was added. The diluted semen was cooled to 5° C over a period of 1½ hr, then held at that temperature for an additional 3 to 6 hr (Exps 1 to 4) or 10 to 12 hr (Exp. 5) before pellet freezing (0·035 ml, Exp. 1; 0·35 ml, Exps 2 to 5) on dry ice. The pellets were thawed in test tubes containing 88·4 mM-sodium citrate (2 : 1, pellets: thawing solution, v/v; Exp. 1) or 80·6 mM-sodium citrate–44·4 mM-glucose solution (1 : 3; Exps 2 to 5) held in a water bath at 37° C. Following thawing in Exps 2 to 5, the semen was centrifuged at 2500 rev/min for 15 min and the supernatant discarded to achieve the concentration of motile spermatozoa required for insemination.

Insemination

Cervical and cervical traction ('deep cervical') inseminations were as described previously (Salamon & Lightfoot, 1967).

In Exp. 2, a series of parameters termed 'classification factors', to distinguish them from true experimental factors, were recorded for each ewe at the time of insemination. These classification factors were: time of detecting ewes in oestrus (18.00 hours or 08.00 hours draft), degree of vaginal constriction (normal, moderate constriction, marked constriction), necessity to drain mucus before insemination (mucus abundant or scarce), number of cervical papillae and the depth to which the inseminating pipette could be inserted into the cervical canal. For the latter observation, inseminating pipettes were calibrated at 1-cm intervals from the tip.

Oxytocin and relaxin

Oxytocin (Syntocinon, Sandoz Australia Pty Ltd) and relaxin (Releasin, Lot 10102.46, 20 mg relaxin reference standard/ml in sesame oil, Warner Lambert Pty Ltd, Australia) were administered by injection into the muscle of the hind leg. Oxytocin was administered at the time of insemination in Exp. 1 and immediately after either the first or second insemination in Exp. 5. In Exp. 4, relaxin was injected immediately after drafting, i.e. between 1 and 12 hr after the onset of oestrus.

Non-returns to service and lambing

The experimental ewe flocks were tested with vasectomized rams for 40 to 50 days after insemination to identify ewes that did not return to service. The non-return data for individual ewes was used to assist in the determination of lambing record (Exps 2 to 5) by udder examination (Dun, 1963) immediately after the conclusion of lambing.

Statistical analyses

The statistical significance of treatment comparisons in all experiments was tested by either analysis of variance, or χ^2 (Claringbold, 1961).

EXPERIMENTAL DESIGNS AND RESULTS

EXPERIMENT 1

The effects of method and time of insemination with frozen ram spermatozoa and the administration of oxytocin on fertility (non-returns to service) were examined in Exp. 1.

The experiment was of factorial design: $2 \times 2 \times 2$; n = 33 or 34, N = 269.

(1) Method of insemination—cervical versus cervical traction

(2) Time of insemination—12 to 24 versus 24 to 36 hr after onset of oestrus

(3) Administration of oxytocin—0 versus 10·0 i.u., i.m. at the time of insemination.

Ewes in oestrus were drafted from the flock twice daily at 06.00 hours and 18.00 hours, and held for either 12 or 24 hr before receiving a single insemination with 0·3 ml of thawed semen containing approximately 120×10^6 motile spermatozoa (0.4×10^9 motile cells/ml). The ewes not returning to service were recorded 38 to 41 days after insemination.

Owing to the sub-optimal methods used for freezing and thawing semen in this experiment (see Materials and Methods), the revival rate was low (25 to

136

30%) and the subsequent *in vitro* viability of the thawed spermatozoa was poor in relation to the semen used in Exps 2 to 5. Partly for this reason, the fertility was very low, with an overall non-return rate of 5·6%. The cervical traction method of insemination, however, resulted in significantly higher fertility than normal cervical insemination (9·7 versus 1·5%, $P<0·01$). There was also an interaction between the administration of oxytocin and method of insemination ($P<0·05$). The percentages of non-returns to service for control and oxytocin-injected ewes were 0·0 and 2·0%, respectively, following cervical insemination, compared with 14·9% and 4·5% after insemination by the cervical traction method. However, in view of the generally low fertility, this interaction is considered to be of little biological significance.

Results were similar whether ewes were inseminated either 12 to 24 or 24 to 36 hr after the onset of oestrus (5·3% and 5·9% respectively). The optimal treatment was insemination by cervical traction 24 to 36 hr after the onset of oestrus without an injection of oxytocin, which resulted in a non-return rate of 17·6%.

EXPERIMENT 2

The effects of inseminate type, and both method of insemination and number of inseminations with frozen ram spermatozoa on lambing were examined in Exp. 2.

The experiment was of factorial design: $3 \times 2 \times 2$; n = 21 to 23, N = 266.

(1) Inseminate type—	Concentration of motile spermatozoa ($\times 10^9$/ml)	Inseminate volume (ml)
(i)	1·5	0·1
(ii)	0·5	0·1
(iii)	0·5	0·3

(2) Method of insemination—cervical versus cervical traction
(3) Number of inseminations—1 versus 2

Ewes in oestrus were drafted from the flock both morning (08.00 hours) and evening (18.00 hours). Ewes detected in oestrus at the evening draft were inseminated for the first time at approximately 09.00 hours the following morning, together with the oestrous ewes from that morning's draft. The second insemination, when required, was performed approximately 12 hr later.

The overall results and χ^2 analysis are presented in Table 1. The concentration of motile spermatozoa in the inseminate had a marked effect on lambing ($P<0·001$). Of the ewes inseminated, 43·8% and 23·7% lambed following insemination with concentrated ($1·5 \times 10^9$/ml) and dilute ($0·5 \times 10^9$/ml) semen respectively. Insemination by the cervical traction method resulted in significantly lower fertility than normal cervical insemination (23·9% versus 37·1%, $P<0·05$). Two inseminations gave a higher lambing rate than a single insemination (38·8% versus 22·6%, $P<0·01$) but there was an interaction ($P<0·05$) between number of inseminations and inseminate type. The effect shown in

TABLE 1

EFFECTS OF TYPE OF INSEMINATE, METHOD OF INSEMINATION AND NUMBER OF INSEMINATIONS WITH FROZEN RAM SPERMATOZOA ON LAMBING

Treatment			No. of ewes		% of ewes lambing
			Inseminated	Lambing	
Type of inseminate					
Concentration of motile spermatozoa ($\times 10^9$/ml)		Volume (ml)			
(i)	1·5	0·1	89	39	43·8
(ii)	0·5	0·1	88	19	21·6
(iii)	0·5	0·3	89	23	25·8
Method of insemination					
Cervical			132	49	37·1
Cervical traction			134	32	23·9
Number of inseminations					
1			137	31	22·6
2			129	50	38·8
Overall			266	81	30·5

Analysis of χ^2

Effect		d.f.	χ^2
Type of inseminate	(A)		
(i) versus (ii and iii)†		1	11·29***
(ii) versus (iii)‡		1	0·38
Method of insemination	(B)	1	5·51*
Number of inseminations	(C)	1	8·16**
A × B		2	1·06
A × C			
(i) versus (ii and iii) × C		1	1·92
(ii) versus (iii) × C		1	4·05*
B × C		1	1·41
A × B × C		2	1·09

† Concentrated versus dilute.
‡ 0·1 ml versus 0·3 ml.
* $P < 0.05$;   ** $P < 0.01$;   *** $P < 0.001$.

TABLE 2

THE RELATIONSHIP BETWEEN THE TYPE OF INSEMINATE AND NUMBER OF INSEMINATIONS ON LAMBING

Type of inseminate		One insemination			Two inseminations		
Concentration of motile spermatozoa ($\times 10^9$/ml)	Volume (ml)	No. of ewes		% of ewes lambing	No. of ewes		% of ewes lambing
		Inseminated	Lambing		Inseminated	Lambing	
1·5	0·1	46	19	41·3	43	20	46·5
0·5	0·1	45	8	17·8	43	11	25·6
0·5	0·3	46	4	8·7	43	19	44·2

Table 2 was due to the comparatively large increase in the proportion of ewes lambing following double insemination with 0·3 ml of dilute $(0·5 \times 10^9$ motile cells/ml) semen. The best treatment was two cervical inseminations with 0·1 ml of concentrated $(1·5 \times 10^9$ motile spermatozoa/ml) semen in which thirteen (61·9%) of the twenty-one inseminated ewes lambed.

Several classification factors were found to be significantly related to fertility. The results suggested the occurrence of an interaction ($\chi^2_1 = 3·71$; $0·05 < P < 0·1$) between time of drafting and number of inseminations on lambing (Table 3). In the single insemination treatment, a higher proportion of evening-draft ewes (inseminated approximately 15 to 25 hr after the onset of oestrus) lambed, compared with the ewes detected in oestrus at the morning draft (inseminated approximately 1 to 15 hr after the onset of oestrus). When a second insemination was given 12 hr after the first, a higher proportion of morning- than evening-draft ewes lambed.

TABLE 3

THE RELATIONSHIP BETWEEN TIME OF DRAFTING AND NUMBER OF INSEMINA-
TIONS ON LAMBING

No. of inseminations	Time of drafting					
	1 hr before first insemination (08.00 hours)			15 hr before first insemination (18.00 hours)		
	No. of ewes		% of ewes lambing	No. of ewes		% of ewes lambing
	Inseminated	Lambing		Inseminated	Lambing	
1 (at 09.00 hours)	77	14	18·2	60	17	28·3
2 (at 09.00 hours and 20.00 hours)	65	29	44·6	64	21	32·8
Overall	142	43	30·3	124	38	30·6

Increases in both the number of cervical papillae ($\chi^2_2 = 10·73$; $P < 0·01$) and depth of insemination (χ^2_1 lin. $= 3·17$; $0·05 < P < 0·1$) were associated with higher lambing rates. Further analysis, however, revealed that these classification factors were not independently distributed. Depth of insemination increased markedly as the number of cervical papillae increased ($\chi^2_4 = 23·26$; $P < 0·001$). The depth of insemination was also related to the degree of vaginal constriction recorded ($\chi^2_4 = 13·74$; $P < 0·01$) due to the fact that a high proportion of ewes with constricted vaginae (indicative of barrenness) permitted only shallow insemination.

Although the cervical traction method of insemination resulted in a poorer lambing than the normal cervical method, it nevertheless achieved a greater depth of insemination. The proportions of ewes in which the depth of insemination was recorded as either less than or equal to 1·0 cm, 1·5 to 2·0 cm, or greater than 2·0 cm, were 27, 60 and 13%, compared with 49, 49 and 2% for the cervical traction and cervical methods of insemination, respectively ($\chi^2_2 = 21·91$; $P < 0·001$).

Perhaps the most important interaction involving classification factors and

139

TABLE 4

THE RELATIONSHIP BETWEEN ABUNDANCE OF MUCUS IN THE VAGINA AND DEPTH OF INSEMINATION ON LAMBING

	Depth of insemination into cervical canal (cm)											
	≤1			>1 to 2			>2			Overall		
	No. of ewes		% of ewes lambing	No. of ewes		% of ewes lambing	No. of ewes		% of ewes lambing	No. of ewes		% of ewes lambing
Vaginal mucus	Inseminated	Lambing		Inseminated	Lambing		Inseminated	Lambing		Inseminated	Lambing	
Not abundant	58	8	13·8	69	26	37·7	10	4	40·0	137	38	27·7
Abundant (required draining before insemination)	43	17	39·5	77	22	28·6	9	4	44·4	129	43	33·3
Overall	101	25	24·8	146	48	32·9	19	8	42·1	266	81	30·5

fertility was that between depth of insemination and abundance of mucus in the vagina ($\chi_2^2 = 8.74$; $P<0.05$; Table 4). Among ewes in which a depth of insemination of only 1 cm or less could be achieved, the lambing rate was much lower when mucus was scarce than when it was abundant (necessitating draining before insemination). Lack of mucus made little difference to fertility among ewes in which insemination depths of greater than 1 cm were achieved.

EXPERIMENT 3

The effects of method of semen collection, inseminate volume and number of inseminations with frozen ram spermatozoa on lambing were examined in Exp. 3.

The experiment was of factorial design: $2 \times 2 \times 2$; n = 27 to 30, N = 231.

(1) Method of semen collection—artificial vagina versus electro-ejaculation
(2) Inseminate volume—0·05 versus 0·15 ml
(3) Number of inseminations—1 versus 2.

The drafting procedure and times of insemination (cervical) were as described for Exp. 2, while the concentration of motile spermatozoa in the thawed semen used for insemination was approximately 1.6×10^9 cells/ml.

TABLE 5

EFFECT OF METHOD OF SEMEN COLLECTION, INSEMINATE VOLUME AND NUMBER OF INSEMINATIONS ON LAMBING

Treatment	No. of ewes		% of ewes lambing
	Inseminated	Lambing	
Method of semen collection			
Artificial vagina	114	55	48·2
Electro-ejaculation	117	52	44·4
P			NS
Inseminate volume			
0·05 ml	116	52	44·8
0·15 ml	115	55	47·8
P			NS
Number of inseminations			
1	116	46	39·7
2	115	61	53·0
P			<0·05
Overall	231	107	46·3

The results are presented in Table 5. Neither method of semen collection, nor decreasing the inseminate volume from 0·15 ml to 0·05 ml significantly affected the lambing results. The proportion of ewes lambing, however, was significantly affected by the number of inseminations. Performing a second insemination approximately 12 hr after the first improved the lambing rate from 39·7% to 53·0% ($P<0.05$). A comparatively high overall lambing rate of 46·3% was obtained and the best treatment was two inseminations with 0·05 ml of semen

141

collected by artificial vagina (seventeen/thirty, 56·7%). There were no inter-actions.

An additional observation was made during the conduct of the experiment. In each of seven ewes, two pellets were thawed in the anterior vagina near the external cervical os. One ewe subsequently lambed.

EXPERIMENT 4

The effect of relaxin on depth of insemination and lambing following insemina-tion with frozen ram spermatozoa was examined in Exp. 4.

Doses of 0, 100, 500 or 2500 guinea-pig units (g-p.u.) of relaxin were admini-stered by intra-muscular injection approximately 12 hr before the first insemina-tion. There were seventeen or eighteen ewes/treatment.

Ewes in oestrus were drafted from the flock at 08.00 hours and 18.00 hours daily and allocated at random to treatments. Morning- and evening-draft ewes were injected with relaxin at 09.00 hours and 21.00 hours respectively (i.e. 1 and 3 hr after drafting) and inseminated (cervical) twice at intervals of 12 and 24 hr after the injection.

The depth to which the inseminating pipette could be inserted into the cervical canal during insemination was influenced neither by the dose of relaxin (1·59, 1·77, 1·56 and 1·71 cm for the 0, 100, 500 and 2500 g-p.u. relaxin treat-ments respectively) nor the time of measurement after its administration (1·63 versus 1·68 cm for the first and second inseminations respectively). Depth of insemination was, however, closely related at both first and second insemina-tions ($\chi_4^2 = 13·79$; $P<0·01$) and was significantly greater in ewes with higher numbers of cervical papillae (linear=linear; $\chi_1^2 = 4·20$; $P<0·05$).

The proportions of ewes lambing in the 0, 100, 500 and 2500 g-p.u. relaxin treatments were 11/17 (64·7%), 9/18 (50·0%), 5/17 (29·4%) and 9/17 (52·9%) respectively. Although the proportion of ewes lambing in the relaxin treatments was lower than that for the control (44·2% versus 64·7%; $0·05<P<0·1$), owing to the low numbers of ewes, conclusions concerning the effect of relaxin on fertility cannot be drawn.

In view of the negative results on depth of insemination presented above, an additional observation was made during the conduct of the experiment. Three ewes were injected with 12,500 g-p.u. of relaxin. The mean depths of cervical penetration at the first and second insemination for these ewes were 1·33 and 1·67 cm respectively, and one of the ewes subsequently lambed.

EXPERIMENT 5

The effects of dose of oxytocin and time of its administration on lambing following insemination with frozen spermatozoa were examined in Exp. 5.

The experiment was of factorial design: 3×2; n = 47 to 50, N = 291.

(1) Dose of oxytocin—0 versus 0·5 versus 5·0 i.u., i.m.

(2) Time of administration of oxytocin—immediately after first versus after second insemination

Ewes in oestrus were drafted from the experimental flock at 08.00 hours daily. All ewes received their first insemination immediately after drafting (approximately 1 to 25 hr after the onset of oestrus) and the second insemination approximately 10 hr later. The concentration of motile spermatozoa in the semen and inseminate volume used for all inseminations (cervical) were approximately 1.5×10^9 cells/ml and 0.1 ml respectively.

Semen used for this experiment was collected from twenty rams of unknown fertility and pellet-frozen under field conditions. The period of 10 to 12 hr for which the diluted semen was stored at 2 to 5° C before freezing was too long for optimal revival rates and subsequent viability of the thawed spermatozoa (Lightfoot & Salamon, 1969). Although there is no direct evidence, it is thought that these factors accounted for the comparatively low overall fertility (27.5% ewes lambing; Table 6) obtained in this experiment compared with that obtained with otherwise similar procedures in Exps 2, 3 and 4.

TABLE 6

LAMBING FOLLOWING THE ADMINISTRATION OF OXYTOCIN AT EITHER THE FIRST OR SECOND INSEMINATION WITH FROZEN RAM SPERMATOZOA

Treatment	No. of ewes		$\%$ of ewes lambing
	Inseminated	Lambing	
Dose of oxytocin (i.u., i.m.)			
0	99	24	24.2
0.5	96	36	37.5
5.0	96	20	20.8
P, 0 versus 0.5 and 5.0			NS
0.5 versus 5.0			<0.01
Time of administration of oxytocin			
After first insemination	144	37	25.7
After second insemination†	147	43	29.3
P			NS
Overall	291	80	27.5

† The second insemination was performed approximately 10 hr after the first insemination.

Injection of 5.0 i.u. oxytocin after insemination resulted in a lower proportion of ewes lambing (20.8%) than occurred in the 0.5 i.u. oxytocin (37.5%) or control (24.2%) treatments. The difference between the former two treatments was statistically significant ($P<0.01$). The lambing rate was not affected by time of administering oxytocin.

DISCUSSION

It would appear from the results of experiments reported here that the methods employed in freezing and thawing ram spermatozoa by the pellet technique are critical for the attainment of satisfactory lambing results. The use of sub-optimal methods of dilution, equilibration and/or thawing in the preparation of semen for Exps 1 and 5 was associated with comparatively poor post-thawing sperm activity and low fertility, although it is likely that other factors were also involved (e.g. one insemination only, low concentration of spermatozoa—Exp. 1; rams of unknown fertility—Exp. 5).

The importance of achieving a high concentration of motile spermatozoa in the inseminate to increase the number of spermatozoa entering the cervix was shown by Lightfoot & Salamon (1970a). In the experiments reported here, the concentration of spermatozoa in the inseminate was found to be a major factor influencing the proportion of ewes lambing. The low fertility observed in Exp. 1, in which semen containing only 0.4×10^9 motile spermatozoa/ml was used, is partly attributable to this factor.

In contrast to the importance of sperm concentration, the inseminate volume appeared to have little effect on the fertility, which is in agreement with the literature for fresh semen (e.g. Robinson, 1956, 1958; Sinclair, 1957; Kuznecov & Kuprijanova, 1961; Jones, Martin & Lapwood, 1969). Reducing the inseminate volume from 0.3 to 0.1 ml in Exp. 2 (0.5×10^9 motile spermatozoa/ml) or from 0.15 to 0.05 ml in Exp. 3 (1.6×10^9 motile spermatozoa/ml) did not significantly affect the lambing rate. It seems likely, at least with ewes in which semen can be deposited into the cervical os, that use of a concentrated inseminate of even less than 0.05 ml may be practical.

The increase in the lambing rate that was achieved by double insemination with frozen semen was greater than that normally reported for inseminations with fresh ram semen (e.g. Sinclair, 1957; Salamon & Robinson, 1962; Dunlop & Tallis, 1964). This is compatible with the evidence (Salamon & Lightfoot, 1967; Mattner, Entwistle & Martin, 1969; Lightfoot & Salamon, 1970a) that infertility following insemination with deep frozen ram semen is associated with a failure of sperm entry and viability within the ewe's genital tract. The magnitude of the response to double insemination with frozen semen, however, seemed to vary according to the characteristics of the inseminate and the timing of insemination in relation to the stage of oestrus of the ewe. In the former case, the increase in fertility was greater with dilute than concentrated semen (Exp. 2, Table 2), and in the latter case, more advantage was gained from performing a second insemination when the first had been given early, rather than towards the middle of oestrus (Table 3). It should be noted, however, that the results reported here conflict with those of other workers who have failed to obtain a fertility response of similar magnitude to double insemination with frozen ram semen (First, Sevinge & Henneman, 1961; Lopatko, 1963; Salamon, 1967).

More experimentation is required before the value of the cervical traction method of insemination can be adequately assessed. In Exp. 1, the results were in favour of this method, but the overall fertility was very low. Normal cervical insemination was superior to the cervical traction method, both in Exp. 2 and in an experiment reported elsewhere (Lightfoot & Salamon, 1970b). Ten En Bon (1965) used frozen semen and reported that 36.0% ewes (201) versus 46.4% ewes (28) lambed following the normal and a 'deep cervical' method of insemination respectively. However, it appears that only those ewes in which a depth of 2 to 5 cm insemination could be achieved were included in the latter treatment.

144

The relationship between depth of insemination and ewe fertility, as indicated in Exp. 2 and reported by Šarapa (1967), is difficult to interpret as insemination depth is closely related to the number of cervical papillae (Exps 2 and 4) which is, in turn, associated with both ewe fertility (Exp. 2) and increasing parity in ewes (Dun, 1955). It is possible that, when using frozen semen, increasing numbers and complexity of the cervical papillae assist in retaining a greater proportion of the inseminate in contact with mucus at the external cervical os, resulting in better penetration of spermatozoa into the cervix. This hypothesis is supported by the observation (Exp. 2) that, in ewes with little mucus and in which only shallow insemination can be achieved, fertility is much reduced.

The hormonal requirements for cervical relaxation in non-pregnant farm animals are not clear. Cervical relaxation has been reported in both swine and cattle with doses of relaxin varying from 500 to 15,000 g-p.u., usually preceded by oestrogen treatment (Graham & Dracy, 1953; Zarrow, Sikes & Neher, 1954; Zarrow, Neher, Sikes, Brennan & Bullard, 1956; Eggee & Dracy, 1966). However, Smith & Nalbandov (1958) found that relaxin injections (750 g-p.u.) did not cause cervical relaxation in sows when given concurrently with oestrogen. Although the range of doses used in the present study with oestrous ewes (100 to 12,500 g-p.u.) seems to be adequate in relation to those used by other workers, there was no visible effect of the hormone on the external os of the cervix, nor was a deeper insemination achieved.

The results of the present experiments do not support the use of oxytocin as an agent to improve fertility in the ewe, contrary to evidence concerning its use in cows (Hays, VanDemark & Ormiston, 1953, 1958; Milovanov & Sergeev, 1961; Milovanov, Sokolovskaja, Korotkov, Gorohov, Masenko, Rymarj & Rahman, 1963; Stepanov, 1964; Masenko, 1966) and sows (Stratman, Self & Smith, 1958; Milovanov & Sergeev, 1961; Sergeev, 1963; Ikoev & Ermakov, 1965). The high doses (5·0 to 10·0 i.u.) used in Exps 1 and 5 depressed ewe fertility, thereby confirming earlier results (Lightfoot & Salamon, 1970a). The lambing rate was slightly higher than controls following the administration of a low dose of oxytocin (0·5 i.u.; Exp. 5) but the effect was not significant, in agreement with experiments conducted with fresh semen by Jones (1968) and Jones et al. (1969). Derjažencev (1966), however, reported increased fertility in a group of ewes inseminated with fresh semen to which a posterior pituitary preparation had been added.

Apart from more recent reports, the literature concerning fertility of deep frozen ram semen has been reviewed by Emmens (1961), Emmens & Robinson (1962) and Sadleir (1966). These reviews point out that critical assessment of many of the reports is difficult as the authors frequently omit essential details concerning the conduct of the experiments. The highest fertility—61 to 66%— has been reported by Mackepladze, Gugušvili, Bregadze & Haratišvili (1960) and by Lopatko (1963)—41 to 67%—but the latter results have not been confirmed (Branny, Pilch & Wierzbowski, 1966; Salamon, 1967; Lopyrin, 1969). Lopyrin reported that the high fertility results claimed by the Soviet workers have subsequently been tested under supervision of a commission and "none of the authors could confirm their own results and obtain a fertility rate higher than 14% after one insemination. Evidently, this was due to the replacement of fertile teaser rams by vasectomized rams. Thus, the possibility of occasional fertilization of ewes by natural mating has been excluded". Aamdal & Andersen (1968) recently reported 62% pregnancy in twenty-six ewes inseminated with semen frozen in straws. Reasonably good results have also been claimed by Kalév & Vénkov (1961; 55% non-returns), Vlachos & Tsakalof (1965; 23 to 56%) and Ten En Bon (1965; 36 to 46%) but the authors have not mentioned what type of teaser rams were used for detection of ewes in oestrus.

Previous publications concerned with ram semen frozen by the pellet method, mentioned earlier, have reported generally low fertility. The comparatively high fertility reported by Lightfoot & Salamon (1970b) has been confirmed in the experiments reported here and a number of factors that may affect the fertility of pellet-frozen ram spermatozoa have been identified. Further development may lie in a critical assessment of the minimum inseminate volume that may be used without reduced fertility to achieve the most economical use of frozen semen.

ACKNOWLEDGMENTS

The authors are indebted to Mr P. G. Walker and Sons of Ledgworth, Yass, N.S.W. (Exps 1 and 4), Mr E. J. Merriman and Mr D. Fletcher of Ravensworth, Yass, N.S.W. (Exp. 2), Mr G. Whitechurch of Brundah, Binalong, N.S.W. (Exp. 3), and Mr P. Nivison of Mirani, Walcha, N.S.W. (Exp. 5), for their generous provision of sheep and facilities.

We wish to thank Professor T. J. Robinson for his comments on the manuscript. The research was aided by grants from the Australian Wool Board and the Australian Research Grants Committee.

Syntocinon and Releasin were generously donated by Sandoz Australia Pty Ltd and Warner Lambert Pty Ltd, Australia, respectively.

REFERENCES

AAMDAL, J. & ANDERSEN, K. (1968) Freezing of ram semen in straws. *Proc. 6th Int. Congr. Anim. Reprod. A.I., Paris,* **2,** 977.

BRANNY, J., PILCH, J. & WIERZBOWSKI, S. (1966) Low temperature freezing of ram semen. II. Diluent trials. *Medycyna wet.* **22,** 290.

CLARINGBOLD, P. J. (1961) The use of orthogonal polynomials in the partition of chi-square. *Aust. J. Statistics,* **3,** 48.

DERJAŽENCEV, V. I. (1966) The use of implementors to increase viscosity and posterior pituitary preparation to increase conception in ewes inseminated cervically. *Sb. nauch. Rab. vses. nauchno-issled. Inst. Zhivot.* No. **3,** 75.

DUN, R. B. (1955) The cervix of the ewe—its importance in artificial insemination of sheep. *Aust. vet. J.* **31,** 101.

DUN, R. B. (1963) Recording the lambing performance of ewes under field conditions. *Aust. J. exp. Agric. Anim. Husb.* **3,** 228.

DUNLOP A. A. & TALLIS, G. M. (1964) The effects of length of oestrus and number of inseminations on the fertility and twinning rate of the Merino ewe. *Aust. J. agric. Res.* **15,** 282.

EGGEE, C. J. & DRACY, A. E. (1966) Histological study of effects of relaxin on the bovine cervix. *J. Dairy Sci.* **49,** 1053.

EMMENS, C. W. (1961) *Dilution, transport and storage of ram semen.* In: Artificial Breeding of Sheep in Australia, p. 118. Proc. Conf. School of Wool Technology, University of N.S.W., Australia.

EMMENS, C. W. & ROBINSON, T. J. (1962) Artificial insemination in the sheep. In: The Semen of Animals and Artificial Insemination. *Tech. Commun. Commonw. Bur Anim. Breed. Genet.* **15,** 205.

FIRST, N. L., SEVINGE, A. & HENNEMAN, H. A. (1961) The fertility of frozen and unfrozen ram semen. *J. Anim. Sci.* **20,** 79.

FRASER, A. F. (1968) Progress in the artificial insemination of sheep with frozen semen. *Proc. 6th Int. Congr. Anim. Reprod. A.I., Paris,* **2,** 1033.

GRAHAM, E. F. & DRACY, A. E. (1953) The effect of relaxin and mechanical dilation on the bovine cervix. *J. Dairy Sci.* **36,** 772.

HAYS, R. L., VANDEMARK, N. L. & ORMISTON, E. E. (1953) Effect of oxytocin and epinephrine on the conception rate of cows. (Abstract). *J. Dairy Sci.* **36,** 587.

HAYS, R. L., VANDEMARK, N. L. & ORMISTON, E. E. (1958) The effect of oxytocin and epinephrine on the conception rate of cows. *J. Dairy Sci.* **41,** 1376.

IKOEV, F. I. & ERMAKOV, N. F. (1965) Effects of pituitrin on conception and fertility of sows. *Svinovodstvo,* **19,** 37. (*Anim. Breed. Abstr.* **34,** No. 2303.)

JONES, R. C. (1968) The fertility of ewes injected with synthetic oxytocin following artificial insemination. *Aust. J. exp. Agric. Anim. Husb.* **8,** 13.

JONES, R. C., MARTIN, I. C. A. & LAPWOOD, K. R. (1969) Studies on the artificial insemination of sheep: The effects on fertility of diluting ram semen, stage of oestrus of the ewe at insemination, and injection of synthetic oxytocin. *Aust. J. agric. Res.* **20,** 141.

KALÉV, G. & VÉNKOV, T. (1961) Sur la méthode de congélation profonde du sperme du taureau, de bélier et de bouc. *Proc. 4th Int. Congr. Anim. Reprod., The Hague,* **4,** 972.

KUZNECOV, M. P. & KUPRIJANOVA, L. P. (1961) Scientific basis for the dose of ram semen required in artificial insemination. *Ovtsevodstvo,* **7**(9), 24.

LIGHTFOOT, R. J. & SALAMON, S. (1969) Freezing ram spermatozoa by the pellet method. II. The effects of method of dilution, dilution rate, glycerol concentration and duration of storage at 5°C prior to freezing on survival of spermatozoa. *Aust. J. biol. Sci.* **22,** 1547.

LIGHTFOOT, R. J. & SALAMON, S. (1970a) Fertility of ram spermatozoa frozen by the pellet method. I. Transport and viability of spermatozoa within the genital tract of the ewe. *J. Reprod. Fert.* **22,** 385.

LIGHTFOOT, R. J. & SALAMON, S. (1970b) Fertility of ram spermatozoa frozen by the pellet method. II. The effects of method of insemination on fertilization and embryonic mortality. *J. Reprod. Fert.* **22,** 399.

LOGINOVA, N. V. & ZELTOBRJUK, N. H. (1968) Test of different methods of freezing semen. *Ovtsevodstvo,* **14**(9), 22.

LOPATKO, M. I. (1963) *Laboratory and field tests on methods of freezing ram semen to* − *196°C.* In: Artificial Insemination of Farm Animals, p. 64. Forrest Steppe Inst. Anim. Breed., Ukrainian S.S.R., Kharkov Book Publisher.

LOPYRIN, A. I. (1969) Recurrent problems of artificial insemination of sheep. *Zhivotnovodstvo, Mosk.* **31** (10), 75.

MACKEPLADZE, I. B., GUGUŠVILI, K. F., BREGADZE, M. A. & HARATIŠVILI, G. (1960) Storage and use of frozen bull and ram semen. *Zhivotnovodstvo, Mosk.* **22**(2), 77.

MASENKO, I. A. (1966) The effect of a preparation of the posterior pituitary and an agent to increase viscosity on semen quality and conception in cows when various dilution rates were used. *Trudy vses. nauchno-issled. Inst. Zhivot.* **29,** 340.

MATTNER, P. E., ENTWISTLE, K. W. & MARTIN, I. C. A. (1969) Passage, survival and fertility of deep-frozen ram semen in the genital tract of the ewe. *Aust. J. biol. Sci.* **22,** 181.

MILOVANOV, V. K. & SERGEEV, N. I. (1961) The simultaneous use of oxytocin—a new method of increasing the effectiveness of artificial insemination of pigs. *Zhivotnovodstvo, Mosk.* **23**(11), 70.

MILOVANOV, V. K., SOKOLOVSKAJA, I. I., KOROTKOV, A. I., GOROHOV, L. N., MASENKO, I. A., RYMARJ, M. A. & RAHMAN, ALI N. E. D. A. (1963) Implementors for increasing conception and fertility in cows and pigs. *Dokl. vses. Akad. sel'.-khoz. Nauk,* **1,** 32. (*Anim. Breed. Abstr.* **32,** No. 2965).

PLATOV, E. M. (1968) The effect of freezing on the content of adenosine polyphosphates in semen. *Ovtsevodstvo,* **14**(8), 14.

ROBINSON, T. J. (1956) The artificial insemination of the Merino sheep following the synchronization of oestrus and ovulation by progesterone injected alone and with pregnant mare serum gonadotrophin (PMS). *Aust. J. agric. Res.* **7,** 194.

ROBINSON, T. J. (1958) Studies in controlled artificial insemination of Merino sheep. *Aust. J. agric. Res.* **9,** 693.

SADLEIR, R. M. F. S. (1966) The preservation of mammalian spermatozoa by freezing. *Lab. Pract.* **15,** 413.

SALAMON, S. (1967) Observations on fertility of ram semen frozen by different methods. *Aust. J. exp. Agric. Anim. Husb.* **7,** 559.

SALAMON, S. & LIGHTFOOT, R. J. (1967) Fertilization and embryonic loss in sheep after insemination with deep frozen semen. *Nature, Lond.* **216,** 194.

SALAMON, S. & ROBINSON, T. J. (1962) Studies on the artificial insemination of Merino sheep. I. The effects of frequency and season of insemination, age of ewe, rams and milk diluents on lambing performance. *Aust. J. agric. Res.* **13,** 52.

ŠARAPA, G. S. (1967) The conception of ewes in relation to insemination technique. *Ovtsevodstvo,* **13**(8), 7.

SERGEEV, N. I. (1963) Results of artificially inseminating pigs when oxytocin and neurotropic substances were used. *Zhivotnovodstvo, Mosk.* 25(2), 76.

SINCLAIR, A. N. (1957) Effect of variation of time of mating, mating frequency and semen dose rate on conception in Merino sheep. *Aust. vet. J.* **33,** 88.

SMITH, J. C. & NALBANDOV, A. V. (1958) The role of hormones in the relaxation of the uterine portion of the cervix in swine. *Am. J. vet. Res.* **19,** 15.

STEPANOV, A. T. (1964) The effect of carbocholine solution and pituitrin on conception in cows. *Zhivotnovodstvo, Mosk.* 26(1), 83.

STRATMAN, F. W., SELF, H. L. & SMITH, V. R. (1958) The effect of oxytocin on fertility in gilts artificially inseminated with a low sperm concentration and semen volume. *J. Anim. Sci.* **18,** 634.

TEN EN BON (1965) Physiological and biochemical characters of semen should be considered in insemination with frozen semen. *Ovtsevodstvo,* **11**(8), 11.

VLACHOS, C. & TSAKALOF, P. (1965) Research on freezing ram semen by means of liquid nitrogen and results of its use in comparison with fresh semen. *Bull. Physiol. Pathol. Reprod. Artif. Insem.* **1,** 71.

VOLKOV, A. S. (1968) Conception in ewes inseminated with deep frozen semen. *Sb. nauch. Rab. vses. Ord. Trud. krans. Znam. nauchno-issled. Inst. Zhivot.* No. **10,** 74. (*Anim. Breed. Abstr.* **37,** No. 593.)

ZARROW, M. X., NEHER, G. M., SIKES, D., BRENNAN, D. M. & BULLARD, J. F. (1956) Dilatation of the uterine cervix of the sow following treatment with relaxin. *Am. J. Obstet. Gynec.* **72,** 260.

ZARROW, M. X., SIKES, D. & NEHER, G. M. (1954) Effects of relaxin on the uterine cervix and vulva of young castrated sows and heifers. *Am. J. Physiol.* **179,** 687.

148

NUMBERS OF SPERMATOZOA IN THE GENITAL TRACT AFTER ARTIFICIAL INSEMINATION OF PROGESTAGEN-TREATED EWES

T. D. QUINLIVAN AND T. J. ROBINSON

INTRODUCTION

Two authors (Hancock, 1962; Anon., 1963) have postulated that an alteration in the pattern of distribution of spermatozoa in the female reproductive tract—and hence in the numbers available for fertilization—may cause the lowered fertility often observed following progestagen treatment for the synchronization of oestrus in sheep and cattle. Experimental evidence for this was presented by the authors (Quinlivan & Robinson, 1967), who found that the pattern of sperm recovery from the Fallopian tubes of the ewe was altered at the first post-withdrawal oestrus following synchronization with intravaginal sponges impregnated with a synthetic fluoro-progestagen (17α-acetoxy-9α-fluoro-11β-hydroxypregn-4-ene-3,20-dione; Cronolone, Searle). Highly significant differences were obtained 24 hr after insemination—the approximate time of ovulation and fertilization in the ewe. Further, the insemination of numbers of spermatozoa within the range 80 to 500 million had little effect on the numbers recovered from the Fallopian tubes or on the fertilization rate of ova.

As the availability of spermatozoa in the Fallopian tubes is determined by the population in other divisions of the tract (Mattner, 1963, 1966), an experiment was conducted at the McCaughey Memorial Institute, Jerilderie, N.S.W., in January and February, 1967, to determine in which segment failure of transport, or survival, takes place, and the time relationships involved.

MATERIALS AND METHODS

Experimental conditions

One hundred and fifty 6-year-old ewes, plus two entire and five vasectomized rams were available. Of these, fifty progestagen-treated and fifty untreated ewes in oestrus were required.

Sixty ewes were treated for 16 days with intravaginal polyurethane sponges, 3·5 cm in diameter and impregnated, in the laboratory, with 30 mg Cronolone (Robinson, 1965).

Fifty-four of the sixty progestagen-treated ewes (90%) exhibited oestrus: fifty were incorporated into the experiment.

Sponges were inserted into the first group of five treated ewes on 18th January and thereafter at the rate of five every other day for 24 days.

The fifty untreated ewes were drawn from the remaining flock of ninety, as they exhibited oestrus.

Vasectomized rams, fitted with sire-sine harnesses and crayons, were joined with the ewes on 3rd February, the day the sponges were withdrawn from the first group of treated animals. Following removal of the sponges, treated and untreated ewes were run together and were inspected for oestrus twice daily at 06.00 and 18.00 hours. Oestrous ewes were inseminated as soon as detected, and were rotationally allocated into one of five groups, depending on the time of slaughter following insemination.

Inseminations were into the external cervical os and, to avoid any undue excitement in the period between insemination and slaughter, the ewes were run in a yard adjacent to the shed.

In order to check the relative times of insemination, examinations were made of the ovaries for follicular activity and of tubal flushings for number and stage of development of ova.

On each occasion of insemination, semen was collected from the two rams by using an artificial vagina. Each sample was examined for density and motility and the ejaculates pooled, the number of spermatozoa/ml estimated by haemocytometer counts, and the volume required to provide 500×10^6 spermatozoa determined. All ewes were inseminated with undiluted semen, all samples of which reached a minimum grading of 4 for both density and motility (Ožin,

1956). This represents semen containing at least 2500×10^6 spermatozoa/ml, of which at least 80% are motile.

Recovery of spermatozoa

Immediately after slaughter at a local abattoir, the abdomen was opened and the genital tract exteriorized. The vagina, cervix, uterus, and isthmus and ampulla of the Fallopian tubes were clamped or ligatured at their respective extremities. The entire tract was then removed and the separate divisions were wrapped in tissue towelling and plastic, and transported to the laboratory. The vagina, cervix, uterus, isthmus and ampulla were dissected free of their attachments and flushed, in that order, into appropriately labelled glass vials with calcium-free Krebs Ringer diluent. A standard method of dissection and flushing was used throughout, and scrupulous attention was paid to the cleanliness of instruments, glassware and personal hygiene. The volume of Krebs Ringer diluent was 10 ml for the vagina, cervix and uterus, and 2 ml, followed by 1·5 ml of air, for the isthmus and ampulla. The two isthmic and two ampullary flushings from the same ewe were pooled. All collections were immediately frozen to -10° C. The time from slaughter to completion of flushing, for any one ewe, ranged from 40 min to 2 hr, depending on the number of genital tracts to be examined.

Two techniques were used for the examination of flushings from the vagina, cervix and uterus.

1. Following thawing and thorough mixing of the 10-ml flushings, six haemocytometers were filled by Pasteur pipette, by the following method. Each chamber of the first haemocytometer was filled from the pipette and the residue returned to the vial. The contents of the vial were re-mixed and a second sample taken, and the procedure repeated until all six haemocytometers were filled. The numbers of spermatozoa in each haemocytometer were counted using the standard technique for white blood cells, with an Improved Neubauer ruling, and the mean for the six haemocytometers was determined. The total volume of the flushing was measured and the estimated number of spermatozoa present in the collection was calculated.

2. When less than twelve spermatozoa were counted in the total of the six haemocytometers (mean <2), a second count was made using the following technique. The flushing was thoroughly mixed and stained with congo red-nigrosin stain (3% w/v congo red; 5% w/v nigrosin; sodium citrate buffer) and 0·3-ml aliquots were deposited on to each of six slides. A 20×40 mm glass coverslip, pillared by Vaseline at six points, was lowered gently on to each sample. The slides were allowed to settle for 15 to 20 min, when the numbers of spermatozoa were counted in four horizontal traverses at $\times 400$ magnification. From these counts the estimated number of spermatozoa in each flushing was calculated.

Flushings from the Fallopian tubes were thawed and stained by adding one drop of congo red-nigrosin stain. After thorough mixing, the total volume of the sample was distributed evenly on to six slides as described above and counted in the same manner. These counts represented one-twelfth of the total area of each slide. Multiplication by twelve of the total number counted on the six

151

slides gave an estimate of the total number of spermatozoa recovered for each ewe.

Experimental design

The experiment had the following factorial design:

Comparison	Description	Factors
1. Synchronization of oestrus	Synchronized versus non-synchronized	2
	(First oestrus) (Untreated)	
2. Time of slaughter (hr after insemination)	1 versus 12 versus 24 versus 36 versus 48 hr	5

$$2 \times 5; \, n = 10; \, N = 100$$

Analyses of variance were conducted on the CSIRO CDC-3600 computer on the $\log_{10}$ numbers of spermatozoa counted (plus one to deal with zero values).

RESULTS

Relative stage of oestrus of synchronized and non-synchronized ewes

Both classes of ewes were inseminated at comparable times, judged by (a) the data for ewes with large follicles or which had ovulated shortly before slaughter (Table 1), and (b) the number of ova recovered. Of sixty-nine ova shed, thirty-seven (59·9%) were recovered, all from the ampulla, nineteen from synchronized and eighteen from untreated ewes. Of these, three were cleaving, at the two-cell stage.

TABLE 1

NUMBER OF EWES WITH LARGE FOLLICLES (>5 MM) OR WHICH HAD
RECENTLY OVULATED WHEN EXAMINED AT SLAUGHTER

Time of slaughter (hr after insemination)	Non-synchronized—controls			Synchronized—first oestrus		
	Total ewes examined	Recently ovulated	With large follicles (>5 mm)	Total ewes examined	Recently ovulated	With large follicles (>5 mm)
1	10	0	8	10	0	8
12	10	1	7	10	1	6
24	10	10	0	10	9	1
36	10	9	1	10	9	1
48	10	10	0	10	10	0
Total	50	30	16	50	29	16

Numbers of spermatozoa recovered

Table 2 shows the estimated mean numbers of spermatozoa recovered from the various divisions of the tract at the five intervals of time. The data are presented in two ways, namely (a) arithmetic means based on the actual numbers counted, and (b) corrected means based on the $\log_{10}$ value for each count, as used in the analysis of variance. These latter values are used for the construction of Text-figs. 1 to 3. Table 3 presents two split-plot analyses of

TABLE 2

ESTIMATED MEAN NUMBERS OF SPERMATOZOA RECOVERED FROM VARIOUS DIVISIONS OF THE GENITAL TRACT AT INTERVALS AFTER INSEMINATION ($\times 10^3$)

Time of slaughter (hr after insemination)	Non-synchronized—controls					Synchronized—first oestrus				
	1 Vagina	2 Cervix	3 Uterus	4 Isthmus	5 Ampulla	1 Vagina	2 Cervix	3 Uterus	4 Isthmus	5 Ampulla
A. Arithmetic means										
1	19087	2531	25	0·24	0·07	22607	2629	22	0·10	0·07
12	2772	1215	58	1·79	0·44	41	2471	28	0·39	0·21
24	1347	1072	88	7·32	0·93	15	153	7	0·72	0·20
36	1151	785	42	1·32	0·25	5	183	7	0·60	0·38
48	164	377	22	0·21	0·42	1	12	5	0·14	0·17
Total	24521	5980	235	10·88	2·11	22669	5448	69	1·95	1·03
B. Corrected (logarithmic) means*										
1	12300	1514	10	0·16	0·05	12300	1350	10	0·04	0·05
12	562	437	17	0·66	0·25	22	562	8	0·27	0·10
24	646	741	62	3·80	0·65	6	81	6	0·36	0·11
36	457	468	28	0·51	0·20	4	31	6	0·24	0·21
48	65	107	12	0·16	0·17	1	9	3	0·08	0·09
Total	14030	3267	129	5·29	1·32	12333	2033	33	0·99	0·56

Total ewes in each treatment group (n) = 10. Columns 1 to 3: haemocytometer counts; columns 4 to 5: slide counts.
* Arithmetic values derived from reconversion of mean log values of individual data.

variance of the data for vagina, cervix and uterus. Analysis 1 is on the mean of six counts for each ewe, and Analysis 2 is on one count only, selected at random. Both analyses are presented as an index of precision of technique. Use of all six counts reduces the error associated with counting by approximately one-half. Thus a six-fold increase in counting time results in only a doubling of precision and does not affect any conclusions.

One hour after insemination, the pattern of distribution of spermatozoa in the genital tract of synchronized and non-synchronized ewes was indistinguishable except for the isthmus, where larger numbers appeared in the latter

TABLE 3

ANALYSES OF VARIANCE OF DATA FOR SPERMATOZOA RECOVERED FROM VAGINA, CERVIX
AND UTERUS FOLLOWING LOG TRANSFORMATION

Source of variation	Degrees of freedom	Mean square†		F†	
		Analysis 1	Analysis 2	Analysis 1	Analysis 2
Main plots					
Synchronization of oestrus	1	88·39	72·80	69·05***	34·34***
Time of flushing	4	75·32	54·03	58·84***	25·49***
Synchronization × time	4	10·28	7·49	8·03***	3·79**
Within (Error)	90	1·28	2·12		
Sub-plots					
Division of tract	2	157·82	110·57	142·18***	59·77***
Division × synchronization	2	24·00	19·13	21·62***	10·34***
Division × time	8	23·54	17·04	21·21***	9·21***
Division × synchronization × time	8	2·54	1·65	2·29*	0·89
Within (Error)	180	1·11	1·85		
Total	299				

* $P<0.05$; ** $P<0.01$; *** $P<0.001$.
† Analysis 1. Total data using means of counts for six slides for each sheep. Analysis 2. Data for one slide selected at random for each sheep.

animals. By 12 hr, distinct differences had become apparent and these increased over the next 12 hr (Text-fig. 1). Overall, there were highly significant differences in numbers of spermatozoa recovered attributable to synchronization of oestrus, time of slaughter and division of the genital tract ($P<0.001$), together with significant interactions between these factors ($P<0.05$ to $P<0.001$).

There was a much more rapid decline with time in the total numbers of spermatozoa recovered from synchronized than from non-synchronized ewes (Text-fig. 2).

Individual analyses of variance of data for each division of the genital tract showed significant effects of synchronization ($P<0.01$ to $P<0.001$) and time of flushing ($P<0.05$ to $P<0.001$) on the numbers of spermatozoa recovered. There were also interactions between synchronization and time which, except in the case of the ampulla, attained significance ($P<0.05$ to $P<0.001$). These characteristics are illustrated in Text-fig. 3.

Vagina. At 1 hr, the numbers of spermatozoa recovered from the vagina of synchronized and non-synchronized ewes were indistinguishable (Table 2).

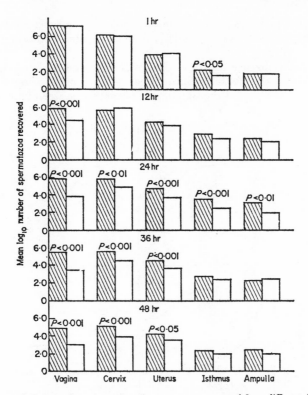

TEXT-FIG. 1. Estimated mean number of spermatozoa recovered from different divisions of the genital tract at each time of slaughter. Hatched columns: non-synchronized (controls); open columns: synchronized.

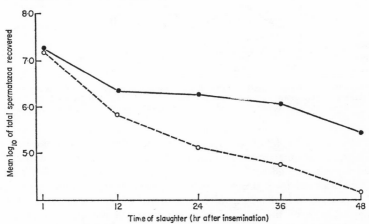

TEXT-FIG. 2. Estimated mean numbers of spermatozoa recovered from the entire reproductive tract at intervals after insemination ($n = 10$, $N = 100$). ●, Non-synchronized (controls); O, synchronized.

155

Thereafter, the numbers fell much more rapidly in the synchronized than in the non-synchronized ewes ($P<0.001$) and the pattern of decline differed significantly (Text-fig. 3a).

In non-synchronized ewes the decline was not simply a linear function of time, as shown by the highly significant quadratic and cubic components of the time effect ($P<0.001$) and the significant interaction between synchronization

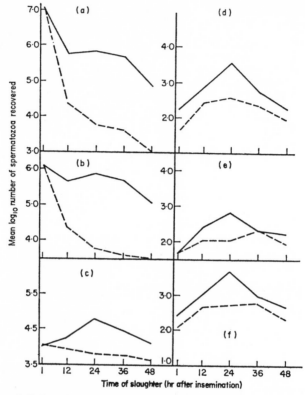

TEXT-FIG. 3. Estimated mean number of spermatozoa recovered from various regions of the tract at intervals after insemination. ———, Non-synchronized (controls); – – – –, synchronized. (a) Vagina; (b) cervix; (c) uterus; (d) isthmus; (e) ampulla; (f) total Fallopian tubes.

and time: quadratic ($P<0.001$). Following an initial large decline between 1 and 12 hr, the numbers remained high until 36 hr after insemination and then fell rapidly again to 48 hr.

In synchronized ewes the pattern was quite different. Following an initial fall, larger than in non-synchronized animals between 1 and 12 hr, there was no maintenance of the vaginal population which continued to fall away, although at a slower rate.

Cervix. Maximum numbers of spermatozoa appeared in the cervical flushings at 1 hr after insemination, when the numbers recovered were indistinguishable

156

in synchronized and non-synchronized ewes (Table 2). Thereafter the pattern was similar for both classes of ewe to that observed for the vagina (Text-fig. 3a, b).

In non-synchronized ewes the cervical population remained high until 36 hr and was still substantial at 48 hr.

In synchronized ewes the numbers fell much more rapidly ($P<0.001$) and, following the initial large fall between 1 and 12 hr, there was no maintenance of a cervical population in the majority of animals.

Uterus. At 1 hr, the numbers of spermatozoa recovered from the uterus of synchronized and non-synchronized ewes were indistinguishable (Table 2), but thereafter the pattern was markedly different (Text-fig. 3c).

In non-synchronized ewes, there was a linear increase in mean numbers until 24 hr after insemination, followed by a linear decline to 48 hr.

In synchronized ewes, there was no such increase to 24 hr, but a steady decline. This difference was significant as shown by the significant quadratic component of the time effect ($P<0.05$) and the significant interaction between synchronization and time: quadratic ($P<0.05$).

Isthmus, ampulla and total Fallopian tubes. The patterns in the segments of the tube were essentially similar and, in the non-synchronized but not in the synchronized ewes, closely mirrored changes in the uterus (Text-fig. 3, d, e, f).

In non-synchronized ewes, there was a linear increase in mean numbers until 24 hr, followed by a linear decline to 48 hr.

In synchronized ewes, there was a slow increase to 36 hr—at which time the numbers were comparable to those in untreated ewes—followed by a decline. The overall difference between the two classes of ewe was highly significant ($P<0.001$) as was the pattern of increase and decrease ($P<0.001$). The different pattern of accumulation of spermatozoa with time after insemination, as shown by the interaction between synchronization and time: quadratic, attained significance in the ampulla and total tube counts ($P<0.05$).

Distribution between animals of numbers of spermatozoa recovered

There was an enormous variation in the number of spermatozoa recovered between animals within treatments. This is reflected by the differences between the arithmetic and logarithmic means in Table 2, and is illustrated for the Fallopian tubes in Text-fig. 4, in which the distributions are essentially similar to those reported earlier (Quinlivan & Robinson, 1967).

Correlations between numbers of spermatozoa recovered from various divisions of the genital tract

Correlation coefficients were calculated for the numbers of spermatozoa recovered from successive regions of the tract at successive time intervals. No clear pattern was evident.

Four positive correlations—two significant ($P\leqslant0.05$) and two near significant ($P<0.10$)—occurred in the non-synchronized ewes. These were vagina-cervix at 1 hr (r = 0.64; $P<0.05$) and 36 hr (r = 0.59; $P<0.10$), cervix-uterus at 12 hr (r = 0.63; $P = 0.05$) and uterus-tubes at 1 hr (r = 0.57; $P<0.10$).

Two negative and one positive correlation—one significant ($P = 0.05$) and two near-significant ($P \leqslant 0.10$)—occurred in the synchronized ewes. These were vagina-cervix at 1 hr (r = -0.61; $P<0.10$), cervix-uterus at 24 hr (r = -0.55; $P = 0.10$) and uterus-tubes at 12 hr (r = 0.63; $P = 0.05$).

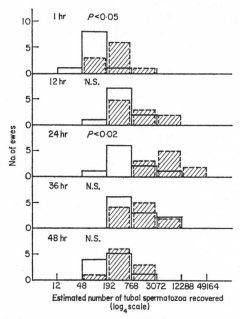

Text-fig. 4. Distribution of number of ewes which yielded tubal spermatozoa, classed into intervals, at 1, 12, 24, 36 and 48 hr after insemination. Hatched columns: non-synchronized (controls); open columns: synchronized.

DISCUSSION

These results confirm and extend those of Quinlivan & Robinson (1967) in that treatment with Cronolone-impregnated intravaginal sponges altered the pattern of sperm transport at the first oestrus following sponge withdrawal, as compared with that in normal oestrous ewes. This difference was not due to insemination at a different stage of oestrus, as the ovarian state at the times of slaughter was indistinguishable between progestagen-treated and untreated control ewes, and the numbers of eggs recovered from the tubes were similar.

The data raise two basic considerations. First, they confirm the effect of progestagen treatment on the transport and survival of spermatozoa in the genital tract, and secondly they elaborate upon the observations of Quinlan, Maré & Roux (1933) and Mattner (1963) on the pattern of sperm transport in the normal cyclic ewe.

Previous studies have indicated that successful sperm transport in the normal ewe is achieved by several events which follow coitus. There is the rapid establishment of reservoirs within the tract, presumably in the cervix (Mattner, 1966), followed by a gradual release of spermatozoa so that adequate numbers are available in the Fallopian tubes at the time of ovulation and fertilization. These concepts have been confirmed in this study with untreated cyclic sheep.

The importance of the vagina as a reservoir has not been defined. Evidence that it may play some role immediately after service has been provided by Krebhiel & Carstens (1939) and Akester & Inkster (1961), who demonstrated that minute jets of radio-opaque fluid passed through the cervices of the rabbit doe during vaginal contractions. Although Noyes, Adams & Walton (1958) and Edgar & Asdell (1960) were unable to confirm this, they reported that radio-opaque media appeared to be forced against the cervix by vaginal contractions.

Our data support the view that the cervix is an important reservoir for spermatozoa. The rapid decline in cervical numbers between 1 and 12 hr after insemination must play a significant role in the establishment of adequate populations in the uterus and Fallopian tubes. Further, the stability of the cervical population between 12 and 24 hr probably involves replenishment over this period, for which the vagina is the only source. During this period the populations in the uterus and the Fallopian tubes are steadily increasing to their maximum at 24 hr.

The establishment of reservoirs other than in the cervix could be anticipated. Table 2 provides evidence that the isthmus may act as a reservoir for the ampulla in the normal ewe. It is estimated that twice as many spermatozoa were present in the isthmus as in the ampulla at 1 hr, and that at 12, 24 and 36 hr this ratio was five, eight and four to one. At 48 hr, the population in the isthmus appeared almost exhausted, probably because of failure of replenishment from the uterus. By analogy with results obtained on laboratory animals, it is generally accepted for the ewe that the isthmus, rather than the utero-tubal junction, constitutes a barrier to the free progression of spermatozoa. This is considered due to the smaller diameter of the lumen, the extensive folding of the mucosa, and the presence of forceful muscular contractions at oestrus (Greenwald, 1963). It is not difficult to visualize that the isthmus may act as a reservoir for the ampulla in much the same manner as does the cervix, and possibly the vagina, for the uterus.

The physiological reasons for the steady increase in sperm numbers in the uterus and the Fallopian tubes up to 24 hr after insemination of the normal oestrous ewe have not been defined. Whatever the mechanisms involved, it appears that maximum chances of successful fertilization depend upon such a pattern of accumulation (Quinlivan & Robinson, 1967).

Spermatozoa may be lost from the genital tract in three ways: first, by voidance to the exterior from the vagina (Blandau & Odor, 1949; Austin, 1957; Reid, 1965a, b); secondly, by passage into the peritoneal cavity (Edgar & Asdell, 1960; Horne & Thibault, 1962; Mattner & Braden, 1963); and thirdly, by phagocytosis within the tract (Chang, 1956; Austin, 1957, 1959; Bedford, 1965; Reid, 1965a; Haynes, 1967).

Comparison of the patterns shown by non-synchronized (normal oestrus) and synchronized ewes (Text-figs. 2 and 3) suggests that two mechanisms are involved in the rapid disappearance of spermatozoa from the vagina within the first 12 hr of insemination. A substantial cervical population is established rapidly, within 1 hr, and, as shown by Text-fig. 2, it is not possible to account for the vaginal loss by compensatory numbers further up the tract. Hence spermatozoa are either destroyed and resorbed *in situ* or are voided to the exterior. It is difficult to attribute the huge difference between the two classes of ewes to differing rates of voidance of unwanted spermatozoa. The inescapable conclusion is that destruction and absorption *in situ* in the vagina is a normal phenomenon and that the rate of such destruction may be greatly accelerated in some physiological states, such as those which exist following synchronization of oestrus.

Most of the loss from the cervix in the normal sheep may be accounted for by forward movement into the uterus in the first stage of the development of the 24-hr peak in sperm population. After 12 hr, the various ways by which spermatozoa may be 'lost' from the genital tract may all play an additive role in the elimination of those spermatozoa not involved in fertilization. The overall effect, as shown in Table 2 and Text-fig. 2, is a linear decline with time in the log number of spermatozoa remaining in the tract.

The failure to demonstrate a meaningful series of significant correlations in the numbers of spermatozoa recovered from various sections of the tract is surprising, and may be related to sample size. The significant correlations between vagina and cervix at 1 hr in normal ewes and between cervix and uterus at 12 hr are almost certainly meaningful and emphasize the importance of the vagina in establishing a large cervical population and of the cervix in establishing an adequate uterine population. The existence of positive, albeit non-significant, correlations between uterine and tubal populations lends support to this concept.

The pattern of sperm transport and survival in the progestagen-treated animal differs substantially from that in the normal ewe. The rate of disappearance of spermatozoa is much more rapid than in normal animals and this process apparently begins within the first 12 hr after service (Table 2, Text-fig. 2). Text-figures 1 and 3 show the development of the pattern of difference. At 1 hr the mean vaginal, cervical and uterine populations are indistinguishable. At 12 hr, the vaginal count in synchronized ewes is significantly depressed and at 24 hr, vaginal, cervical, uterine and tubal counts are all down significantly. The inability of the treated animals to maintain an adequate cervical population between 12 and 24 hr appears to be a key factor in the failure to establish and maintain an adequate uterine and tubal population at 24 hr. This excessive disappearance of spermatozoa is due, presumably, to death and resorption rather than to any significant caudal or cranial shift and subsequent loss.

Smallwood & Sorensen (1967) and Quinlivan (1967) demonstrated apparent histological abnormalities in the endometria of progestagen-treated cattle and sheep at the first post-withdrawal oestrus. These were characterized by the persistence of degenerative changes which seemingly follow the waning of the corpus luteum in the normal cycle or the sudden cessation of exogenous progestagen treatment. Further, the mobilization of excessive numbers of polymorphonuclear leucocytes underlying the basement membrane, was also demonstrated. Moore & Robinson (1967) reported a high density of Corynebacteria and gram-negative bacilli in intravaginal sponges, particularly those inserted without any bactericide. Vaginal smears from treated ewes had an abundant flora, the nature of which was affected by the use of bactericides with the sponges. Subsequently, Quinlivan (1967) found high concentrations of *Corynebacterium pyogenes* and coliforms in the cervical mucus of treated sheep, due presumably to continual contamination of the sponge string by faeces and urine and the retention of an intravaginal foreign body. This may contribute to the depletion in sperm numbers in the genital tract, and particularly in the vagina.

Variable fertility is a feature of all forms of progestagen treatment for the control of the oestrous cycle. However, it is not an invariable feature and satisfactory fertility has been reported in some tests involving the use of intravaginal sponges (Robinson, 1965; Robinson, Quinlivan & Baxter, 1968). One factor appears to be the amount of progestagen absorbed, indicating the need for further studies on the effect of endocrine status at oestrus on the pattern of sperm transport and survival. It should be possible to manipulate this status, and hence the pattern of accumulation of spermatozoa in the Fallopian tubes, so as to increase or decrease the chances of fertilization without affecting ovulation.

ACKNOWLEDGMENTS

Grateful acknowledgment is made to the Trustees of the McCaughey Memorial Institute, Jerilderie, for the provision of experimental animals and facilities; to Mr A. D. Barnes and Miss M. A. Hutchins for field and technical assistance; and to the management and staff of the abattoir at Finley, N.S.W.

One author (T.D.Q.) was holder of a Sir Walter Mulholland Fellowship awarded by the New Zealand University Grants Committee, Wool Board and Romney Association. Experimental materials were generously supplied by G. D. Searle and Co. (Aust.), Sydney. The work was supported by a grant from the Australian Research Grants Committee.

REFERENCES

AKESTER, A. R. & INKSTER, I. J. (1961) Cineradiographic studies of the genital tract of the rabbit. *J. Reprod. Fert.* 2, 507.

ANON. (1963) *Ann. Rep. C.S.I.R.O., Anim. Res. Lab., Div. Anim. Physiol.* 71.

AUSTIN, C. R. (1957) Fate of spermatozoa in the uterus of the mouse and the rat. *J. Endocr.* 14, 335.

AUSTIN, C. R. (1959) Entry of spermatozoa into the Fallopian tube mucosa. *Nature, Lond.* 183, 908.

BEDFORD, J. M. (1965) Effect of environment on phagocytosis of rabbit spermatozoa. *J. Reprod. Fert.* 9, 249.

BLANDAU, R. J. & ODOR, D. L. (1949) The total number of spermatozoa reaching various segments of the reproductive tract in the female albino rat at intervals after insemination. *Anat. Rec.* 103, 93.

CHANG, M. C. (1956) Reaction of the uterus on spermatozoa in the rabbit. *Annali Ostet. Ginec.* 78, 74.

EDGAR, D. G. & ASDELL, S. A. (1960). Spermatozoa in the female genital tract. *J. Endocr.* 21, 321.

GREENWALD, G. S. (1963) *In vivo* recording of intralumenal pressure changes in the rabbit oviduct. *Fert. Steril.* 14, 666.

HANCOCK, J. L. (1962) Fertilization in farm animals. *Anim. Breed. Abstr.* 30, 285.

HAYNES, N. B. (1967) *The influence of the uterine environment on the phagocytosis of spermatozoa.* In: Reproduction in the Female Mammal, p. 500. Proc. 13th Easter School, Univ. Nottingham, 1966. Eds. G. E. Lamming and E. C. Amoroso. Butterworths, London.

HORNE, H. W. & THIBAULT, J. (1962) Sperm migration through the female reproductive tract. *Fert. Steril.* 13, 135.

KREBHIEL, R. H. & CARSTENS, H. P. (1939) Roentgen studies of the mechanism involved in sperm transportation in the female rabbit. *Am. J. Physiol.* 125, 571.

MATTNER, P. E. (1963) Spermatozoa in the genital tract of the ewe. II. Distribution after coitus. *Aust. J. biol. Sci.* 16, 688.

MATTNER, P. E. (1966) Formation and retention of the spermatozoan reservoir in the cervix of the ruminant. *Nature, Lond.* 212, 1479.

MATTNER, P. E. & BRADEN, A. W. H. (1963) Spermatozoa in the genital tract of the ewe. I. Rapidity of transport. *Aust. J. biol. Sci.* 16, 473.

MOORE, N. W. & ROBINSON, T. J. (1967) *A comparison of progesterone-impregnated and non-impregnated intravaginal sponges treated with several bactericides.* In: The Control of the Ovarian Cycle in the Sheep, p. 102. Ed. T. J. Robinson. Sydney University Press, Sydney.

NOYES, R. W., ADAMS, C. E. & WALTON, A. (1958) Transport of spermatozoa into the uterus of the rabbit. *Fert. Steril.* 9, 288.

OŽIN, F. V. (1956) *Artificial insemination in sheep.* Sel'khozgiz., Leningrad.

QUINLAN, J., MARÉ, G. S. & ROUX, L. L. (1933) A study of the duration of motility of spermatozoa in the different divisions of the reproductive tract of the Merino ewe. *Onderstepoort J. vet. Sci.* 1, 135.

QUINLIVAN, T. D. (1967) *Sperm transport and fertilization in normal and progestagen-treated ewes.* Ph.D. thesis, University of Sydney.

QUINLIVAN, T. D. & ROBINSON, T. J. (1967) *The number of spermatozoa in the Fallopian tubes of ewes at intervals after artificial insemination following withdrawal of SC-9880 impregnated intravaginal sponges.* In: The Control of the Ovarian Cycle in the Sheep, p. 177. Ed. T. J. Robinson. Sydney University Press.

REID, B. L. (1965a) The fate of uterine spermatozoa in the mouse *post coitum. Aust. J. Zool.* 13, 189.

REID, B. L. (1965b) The fate of isotope labelled uterine spermatozoa in the mouse *post coitum. Aust. J. Zool.* 13, 525.

ROBINSON, T. J. (1965) Use of progestagen-impregnated sponges inserted intravaginally or subcutaneously for the control of the oestrous cycle in the sheep. *Nature, Lond.* 206, 39.

ROBINSON, T. J., QUINLIVAN, T. D. & BAXTER, C. (1968) The relationship between dose of progestagen and method of preparation of intravaginal sponges on their effectiveness for the control of ovulation in the ewe. *J. Reprod. Fert.* 17, 471.

SMALLWOOD, C. M. & SORENSEN, A. M. (1967) Histological changes in the cow following progestins. *J. Anim. Sci.* 26, 951.

STUDIES ON THE NUMBER OF EWES JOINED PER RAM FOR FLOCK MATINGS UNDER PADDOCK CONDITIONS

I. MATING BEHAVIOUR AND FERTILITY

By R. J. LIGHTFOOT and J. A. C. SMITH

I. INTRODUCTION

There are few reports in the literature concerning the effect of varying the number of ewes joined per ram on flock fertility. Terrill and Stoehr (1939) found no relationship between fertility and the number of ewes joined per ram for pen matings, and in New Zealand Haughey (1959) came to the conclusion that one ram per 100 ewes is more than adequate provided the flocks are run in small paddocks. Extensive trials by Edgar (1965), also in that country, showed no difference in ewe fertility following flock matings at either one, two, or three rams per 100 ewes joined. These results are supported by the observation that the ram is capable of serving a large number of ewes per day, and by evidence (Quinlan, Maré, and Roux 1933; Starke 1949) that sperm can survive for long periods in the cervix, so that a single service within fairly wide time limits during oestrus may result in good fertility (Green 1947).

Whereas such evidence indicates that under certain conditions one ram per 100 ewes can be sufficient, this may not be so in more severe environments. The experiments reported here were undertaken to examine the relationship between number of ewes joined per ram and resultant flock fertility under "wheat-belt" conditions in south Western Australia.

163

TABLE 1

PRINCIPAL FEATURES OF DESIGN AND CONDUCT FOR ALL EXPERIMENTS

Experiment No.:	1	2	3	4	5	6
Design	Factorial (2×3)	Single classification	Factorial (3×4)	Factorial $(2 \times 2 \times 2)$	Single classification	Single classification
Treatments	Rams/ewes: (1)† 1/100 (300)‡ (2)† 1/40 (120) Ram liveweight: Low (140) Medium (140) High (140)	Rams (1½ years old)/ewes: (1)† 1/100 (300) (2)† 1/40 (120) Rams (2½ years old)/ewes: (3)† 1/40 (120)	Rams/ewes: (1)† 1/100 (400) (2)† 1/50 (200) (3)† 1/25 (100) Sperm/ejaculate: $4 \cdot 0 \times 10^9$ (175) $3 \cdot 4 \times 10^9$ (175) $2 \cdot 8 \times 10^9$ (175) $2 \cdot 2 \times 10^9$ (175)	Rams/ewes: (1)† 1/50 (800) (2)† 1/25 (800) Age of rams: 1½ years (800) 3½–5½ years (800) Age of ewes: 1½ years (800) 3½–5½ years (800)	Rams/ewes: (1)† 1/50 (200) (2)† 1/25 (200)	Rams/ewes: (1)† 1/50 (200) (2)† 1/25 (200)
Total no. of rams Total no. of ewes	6 420	9 540	12 700	48 1600	12 400	12 400
Age of rams Age of ewes	1½ years 3–6 years	1½ v. 2½ years 3–6 years	1½ years 2–6 years	1½ v. 2½–5½ years 1½ v. 2½–5½ years	1½–5½ years 1½–5½ years	1½–5½ years 4–7 years
Ram joining	Individual	Group	Individual	Group	Group	Group
Date of joining Period of joining	14.ii.1963 6 weeks	18.ii.1964 6 weeks	3.iii.1965 6 weeks	Feb. 1966 8 weeks	Feb. 1966 8 weeks	Feb. 1966 8 weeks
Location	Wongan Hills	Wongan Hills	Wongan Hills	Merredin	Merredin	Newdegate

† Treatment No. referred to in text.   ‡ Number of ewes per treatment given in parenthesis.

II. Materials and Methods

The principal features of design and conduct for each experiment are shown in Table 1. Other relevant details are given below.

(a) Location and Sheep

Experiments 1 to 3 were conducted on an Agricultural Research Station at Wongan Hills, experiments 4 and 5 on a private property near Merredin, and experiment 6 on a Research Station at Newdegate in south Western Australia. A Mediterranean climate is experienced at all three locations, with c. 75% of the annual average rainfall of 12–15 inches falling in the period May to October. Throughout the summer months maximum ambient temperatures are usually high and frequently rise above 100°F, especially during the months of January and February. Pastures at Wongan Hills and Newdegate are sown to subterranean clover (*Trifolium subterraneum* L. cv. Dwalganup), whereas those at Merredin are sown to barrel medic (*Medicago tribuloides* Desr. cv. Cyprus).

The animals used in experiments 1, 2, 3, and 6 were South Australian strain Merinos whereas those in experiments 4 and 5 were of Peppin origin. Rams in experiments 1, 2, 3, and 6 were all drawn from one stud and were, therefore, of similar pedigree and rearing. All rams received feed supplements and were in good condition prior to joining, the 1½-year-olds ranging from 110 to 140 lb liveweight.

The ewes in experiment 6 were drawn from a flock of poor fertility due to prolonged grazing on oestrogenic pastures (Bennetts, Underwood, and Shier 1946).

(b) Allocation to Treatments and Treatment prior to Joining

In experiment 1, rams were allocated to treatments according to pre-joining liveweight. The six rams were divided, two rams each to "low" (114 lb), "medium" (127 lb), and "high" (140 lb) liveweight groups. Within each group the rams were then randomly allocated to either the 100 or 40 ewes per ram treatment. A similar procedure was used in experiment 3, except that the index for stratification prior to random allocation to the three main treatments was mean total sperm per ejaculate (4·0, 3·4, 2·8 *v.* 2·2×10⁹) from four collections (artificial vagina) made prior to joining. In experiments 2, 4, 5, and 6, rams within each age group were randomly allocated to treatments, as were the ewes in all experiments.

In experiments 3, 4, and 5 the rams were given 10⁶ i.u. of vitamin A 6 weeks allocatedprior to and again immediately before the start of joining.

(c) Mating Observations and Treatment during Joining

In experiments 1, 2, and 3 ewe service records were obtained by inspection for rump marks (Sire-sine ram harness; Radford, Watson, and Wood 1960) at intervals of 7 days, 14 days, and 1 day respectively. Additional data were obtained in experiment 2 by fitting crayons of different colour (red, blue, or green) to individual rams within treatments. Records for individual ewes were kept only in treatment 2.

The rams in experiments 1, 2, and 3 were removed from their ewe flocks for periods of 2–3 hr on several occasions throughout joining for the purpose of semen collection and evaluation (Lightfoot 1968).

Large paddocks (100–200 acres) were used to graze each treatment flock during joining in all experiments except No. 3. On this occasion each group ran on a 6 acre paddock and were given supplements of wheat grain and oaten hay to ensure similar levels of nutrition.

(d) Lambing Observations

All treatment groups were run as one flock at the conclusion of joining until 2 weeks prior to lambing, when the original groups were re-established. In experiments 1, 2, and 3 each ewe was identified by large numbers branded on each side, and the groups were inspected twice daily to record the date each ewe lambed and the number of lambs born. The total number of lambs born, lamb deaths, and lambs marked were obtained for each group in experiments 4, 5, and 6.

(e) Statistical Analyses

In experiments 1, 2, and 3 main effects and their interactions for both service and lambing data were examined by the chi-square method. The effects of treatments on lambing performance in experiment 4 were tested by analysis of variance after rectangular transformation of the data (Biggers 1951; Claringbold and Emmens 1961). In this case individual ewes were scored according to the number of lambs born (0, 1, 2, or 3) so that total treatment scores corresponded to the total number of lambs born in those treatments.

III. Results

(a) Experiment 1

(i) Number and Proportion of Ewes Served

The rams in treatment 1 (one ram to 100 ewes) served more ewes during each of the 6 weeks of joining than did those in treatment 2 (one ram to 40 ewes; Fig. 1(a)). Only 57% of the ewes in treatment 1, however, were served during the first 2 weeks of joining, compared with 77% of treatment 2 ewes during the same period (Fig. 1(b); $\chi_1^2 = 14 \cdot 63$; $P < 0 \cdot 001$). During the last 3 weeks of joining a higher proportion of ewes were served in treatment 1 owing to a greater number of ewes returning to service. At the conclusion of joining, 22 ewes (7·3%) in treatment 1 had not been served throughout the 6 week period, compared with two ewes (1·6%) in treatment 2 (Fig. 1(c); $\chi_1^2 = 4 \cdot 07$; $P < 0 \cdot 05$).

(ii) Conception Rates and Lambing Results

The ewe "conception rate" (ewes lambing/ewes served) was considerably higher in treatment 2 during the first 3 weeks of joining than in treatment 1 (Fig. 3(a)). The conception rate for treatment 2 was lower during the last 3 weeks of joining, but most of the ewes served during this period were returns to service. It was observed that the conception rate for first services was much higher than that for returns to service (71% v. 34%) in treatment 2 but there was little difference in treatment 1 (49% v. 42%).

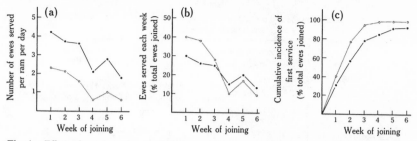

Fig. 1.—Effect of number of ewes joined per ram on various observations during joining: experiment 1. ● Treatment 1 (1 ram/100 ewes). ○ Treatment 2 (1/40).

Joining 40 ewes per ram resulted in a significantly higher proportion of ewes lambing ($P < 0.001$) and a higher proportion of ewes producing twins ($P < 0.05$) to ewes joined (Table 2). Treatment 2 produced 27% more lambs born to ewes joined than treatment 1.

Highly significant differences in lambing performance ($P < 0.001$) were also found between ram liveweight groups, the medium weight rams being more fertile than either the low or the high group.

TABLE 2

EFFECT OF NUMBER OF EWES JOINED PER RAM ON FERTILITY, INDIVIDUAL RAM MATINGS: EXPERIMENT 1

Percentage of:	Ewes Lambing†		Ewes with Twins†		Lambs Born†	
Ratio rams/ewes:	1/100	1/40	1/100	1/40	1/100	1/40
Ram liveweights:						
"Low" group	53	87	6	16	59	103
"Medium" group	83	92	12	19	95	111
"High" group	59	77	8	13	67	90
Treatment means	65	85	9	16	74	101

	Proportion of:	Ewes Lambing	Ewes Twinning
100 v. 40 ewes joined per ram:	$\chi_1^2 =$	18·01***	4·05*
Between-ram liveweight groups:	$\chi_2^2 =$	22·27***	2·83

* $P < 0.05$.   *** $P < 0.001$.   † Percentage in relation to number of ewes joined.

(b) Experiment 2

(i) Mating Records

Many more ewes were served during the first 2 weeks of joining in treatment 1 than in treatment 2 (218 v. 85), but the proportions of ewes served during the same period were similar (73% v. 71%).

167

The $2\frac{1}{2}$-year-old rams (treatment 3) served a significantly higher proportion of ewes (83% $v.$ 71%; $\chi_1^2 = 3\cdot94$; $P<0\cdot05$) during the first 2 weeks of joining than the $1\frac{1}{2}$-year-old rams (treatment 2).

TABLE 3

EFFECT OF NUMBER OF EWES JOINED PER RAM WITH GROUP RAM MATINGS ON ASPECTS OF MATING BEHAVIOUR: EXPERIMENT 2

Treatment	Percentage of Ewes Served by			Mean Number of Rams Serving Oestrous Ewes		
	1 Ram only	2 Rams	All 3 Rams	Weeks 1–2 of Joining	Weeks 3–4 of Joining	Weeks 5–6 of Joining
(1) 3 rams/300 ewes	31	50	19	1·80	1·92	2·02
(2) 3 rams/120 ewes	20	50	30	1·88	2·39	2·42
	$\chi_2^2 = 10\cdot65$**			Between treatments: $\chi_1^2 = 7\cdot34$** Between periods of mating: $\chi_2^2 = 11\cdot46$**		

** $P<0\cdot01$.

Most oestrous ewes in treatments 1 and 2 were served by two of the possible three rams (Table 3). Of the remaining oestrous ewes, a larger proportion was served by one ram in treatment 1 than in treatment 2, whereas a greater proportion of ewes was served by three rams in treatment 2 than in treatment 1 ($\chi_2^2 = 10\cdot65$; $P<0\cdot01$).

TABLE 4

EFFECT OF NUMBER OF EWES JOINED PER RAM AND RAM AGE ON FLOCK FERTILITY, GROUP RAM MATINGS: EXPERIMENT 2

Treatment	Percentage Ewes Lambing†	Percentage Ewes with Twins†	Percentage Lambs Born†	Percentage Lambs Marked†
(1) 3 $1\frac{1}{2}$-year-old rams/ 300 ewes	78	8	86	74
(2) 3 $1\frac{1}{2}$-year-old rams/ 120 ewes	89	13	102	93
(3) 3 $2\frac{1}{2}$-year-old rams/ 120 ewes	91	19	110	100

Proportion of ewes lambing:
Treatment 1 $v.$ treatment 2: $\chi_1^2 = 6\cdot29$ ($P<0\cdot05$)
Treatment 2 $v.$ treatment 3: $\chi_1^2 = 2\cdot27$ NS
Proportion of ewes with twins:
Treatment 1 $v.$ treatment 2: $\chi_1^2 = 1\cdot10$ NS

† Percentage in relation to the number of ewes joined.

More rams served each oestrous ewe in treatment 2 than in treatment 1 ($P<0\cdot01$; Table 3), while in both treatments the mean number of rams serving each oestrous ewe increased as joining progressed ($P<0\cdot01$).

(ii) *Lambing Results*

Joining three rams to 120 ewes (treatments 2 and 3) resulted in a significantly higher proportion of ewes lambing (Table 4; $P < 0.05$) and more ewes giving birth to twins ($0.1 < P < 0.2$) than resulted from joining three rams to 300 ewes (treatment 1). Although joining $2\frac{1}{2}$-year-old rams (treatment 3) resulted in both more ewes lambing and a greater number of ewes giving birth to twins than with $1\frac{1}{2}$-year-old rams (treatment 2), the effects were not statistically significant.

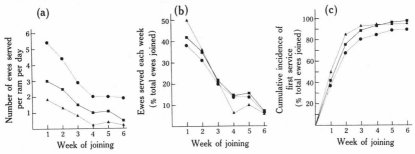

Fig. 2.—Effect of number of ewes joined per ram on various observations during joining: experiment 3. ● Treatment 1 (1 ram/100 ewes). ■ Treatment 2 (1/50). ▲ Treatment 3 (1/25).

(c) *Experiment 3*

(i) *Number and Proportion of Ewes Served*

As in experiment 1, the mean number of ewes served per ram per day increased as the ratio of ewes per ram increased; however, the proportion of ewes served during the first 14 days of joining decreased (Fig. 2(a), (b)). After 14 days of joining the proportions of ewes in treatments 1, 2, and 3 that had been served were 68, 76, and 85% respectively (Fig. 2(c)), the difference between treatments being significant ($\chi_2^2 = 12.33$; $P < 0.01$).

At the conclusion of the 6 week joining period a significantly greater proportion of ewes remained unmated in treatment 1 than in treatments 2 and 3 (10% v. 2% v. 5%; $\chi_2^2 = 13.17$; $P < 0.01$).

(ii) *Conception Rates and Lambing Results*

Ewe "conception rate" (ewes lambing/ewes served) during the first 3 weeks of joining increased significantly as the number of ewes joined per ram decreased (Fig. 3(b)).

Increasing the percentage of rams for mating resulted in improved lambing results: 64, 75, and 91% of the ewes joined in treatments 1, 2, and 3 respectively gave birth to lambs ($P < 0.001$; Table 5). Differences in the proportion of ewes lambing between the four ram groups (pre-joining total sperm per ejaculate) were also statistically significant ($P < 0.001$), group 3 giving the highest and group 4 the lowest level of ewe fertility.

The proportion of ewes giving birth to twins in relation to both the number of ewes joined and the number of ewes lambing also increased progressively from treatment 1 to 3 ($P < 0.01$ and $0.1 < P < 0.2$ respectively). The mean percentages of lambs born to ewes joined were respectively 71, 90, and 110% in treatments 1, 2, and 3.

TABLE 5

EFFECT OF NUMBER OF EWES JOINED PER RAM ON FERTILITY, INDIVIDUAL RAM MATINGS: EXPERIMENT 3

Percentage of:	Ewes Lambing†			Ewes with Twins†			Lambs Born†			Lambs Marked†		
Ratio rams/ewes:	1/100	1/50	1/25	1/100	1/50	1/25	1/100	1/50	1/25	1/100	1/50	1/25
Ram group (sperm/ejaculate):‡												
(1) $4 \cdot 0 \times 10^9$	83	54	88	15	12	24	98	66	112	91	54	108
(2) $3 \cdot 4 \times 10^9$	55	76	92	8	14	24	63	90	116	55	76	96
(3) $2 \cdot 8 \times 10^9$	78	88	92	6	18§	13	84	108	104	78	96	92
(4) $2 \cdot 2 \times 10^9$	37	82	92	3	14	17	40	96	108	38	78	92
Treatment means	64	75	91	8	15	20	71	90	110	66	76	97
Ewes joined per ram	$\chi^2_2 = 32 \cdot 31$***			$\chi^2_2 = 12 \cdot 19$**								
Between ram groups	$\chi^2_3 = 30 \cdot 18$***			$\chi^2_3 = 5 \cdot 08$								

** $P < 0 \cdot 01$.   *** $P < 0 \cdot 001$.   † Percentage in relation to number of ewes joined.

‡ Pre-mating mean total sperm per ejaculate.   § Includes one set of triplets.

(iii) *Relationship between Number of Ewes Served and Ewe Conception Rate: Experiments 1 and 3*

The relationship between number of ewes served per ram each week and resultant ewe conception rate during the first 3 weeks of joining in both experiments 1 and 3 was examined by regression analysis. As neither the regressions for individual

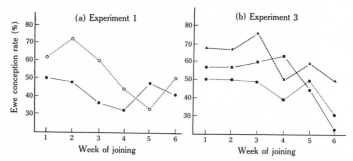

Fig. 3.—Effect of number of ewes joined per ram on ewe "conception rate" (ewes lambing/ewes served) during joining: experiments 1 and 3. ● Treatment 1 (1 ram/100 ewes). ○ Treatment 2 (1/40). ■ Treatment 2 (1/50). ▲ Treatment 3 (1/25).

treatments within experiments nor those for experiments 1 and 3 were significantly different, the overall regression ($P < 0 \cdot 05$), shown below, was calculated.

Percentage ewe conception = $68 \cdot 58 - 0 \cdot 56$ (no. of ewes served per ram per week),

$$S.E. = \pm 5 \cdot 19, \ \pm 0 \cdot 24;$$

$$r = -0 \cdot 31 \ (n = 54, \ P < 0 \cdot 05).$$

Although the limits of error on this relationship are wide, owing to the large variation in fertility between individual rams, it provides additional support for the existence of an inverse relationship between ewe fertility and number of ewes joined per ram.

(d) Experiment 4

Highly significant effects on the number of lambs born were obtained for both the number of ewes joined per ram (Table 6; $P < 0.001$) and age of rams ($P < 0.001$). These effects, however, must be interpreted in relation to the significant ewe/ram ratio × age of rams interaction ($P < 0.001$). Decreasing the number of ewes

TABLE 6

ANALYSIS OF VARIANCE OF NUMBER OF LAMBS BORN PER EWE, MADE BY USING THE RECTANGULAR TRANSFORMATION: EXPERIMENT 4

Factors	D.F.	Mean Square
Number of ewes joined per ram (A)	1	231·1***
Age of rams (B)	1	378·1***
Age of ewes (C)	1	190·1***
A × B	1	253·1***
A × C	1	66·1***
B × C	1	0·1
A × B × C	1	15·1
Error†	∞	4·104

*** $P < 0.001$.

† Theoretical variance: No. of ewes per cell = 200.

joined per ram from 50 to 25 resulted in higher lambing percentages in the case of $1\frac{1}{2}$-year-old rams, but not with $3\frac{1}{2}$–$5\frac{1}{2}$-year-old rams. The $1\frac{1}{2}$-year-old rams were as fertile as the older rams when joined at 25 ewes per ram but were less fertile when 50 ewes were joined per ram (Table 7, Fig. 4).

TABLE 7

INTERACTION BETWEEN NUMBER OF EWES JOINED PER RAM AND BOTH AGE OF RAM AND AGE OF EWE ON FLOCK FERTILITY, GROUP MATINGS: EXPERIMENT 4

(a) % Lambs Born to Ewes Joined   (b) % Lambs Marked to Ewes Joined

Number of Ewes Joined per Ram	Age of Rams (years) $1\frac{1}{2}$	$3\frac{1}{2}$–$5\frac{1}{2}$	Age of Ewes (years) $1\frac{1}{2}$	$2\frac{1}{2}$–$5\frac{1}{2}$	Treatment Means	Age of Rams (years) $1\frac{1}{2}$	$3\frac{1}{2}$–$5\frac{1}{2}$	Age of Ewes (years) $1\frac{1}{2}$	$2\frac{1}{2}$–$5\frac{1}{2}$	Treatment Means
50 (200 ewes/4 rams)	79	91	84	86	85	68	79	72	74	73
25 (200 ewes/8 rams)	90	91	87	94	90	80	80	76	84	80
Treatment means	84	91	85	90	88	74	79	74	79	77

Maiden ewes $1\frac{1}{2}$ years old produced less lambs than $2\frac{1}{2}$–$5\frac{1}{2}$-year-old previously mated ewes ($P < 0.001$), the effect being more marked when ewes were joined at the rate of 25 ewes than at 50 ewes per ram (Tables 6, 7; interaction, $P < 0.001$). There was no evidence of an interaction between age of rams and age of ewes.

The treatment effects and interactions for number of lambs marked were similar to those for number of lambs born.

171

The numbers of lambs born and lambs marked in experiments 5 and 6 are shown in Table 8. In both experiments more lambs were born and marked in the flocks joined at the rate of 25 ewes per ram, the difference being particularly large in

TABLE 8

EFFECT OF NUMBER OF EWES JOINED PER RAM ON FLOCK FERTILITY, GROUP MATINGS: EXPERIMENTS 5 AND 6

Observation	Experiment 5		Experiment 6	
	Number of Ewes Joined per Ram			
	50†	25‡	50†	25‡
Percentage of lambs born to ewes joined	77	90	52	73
Percentage of lambs marked to ewes joined	73	78	38	60

† Four rams/200 ewes.   ‡ Eight rams/200 ewes.

experiment 6, where the fertility of the ewes was lower owing to clover disease. Weekly lambing observations showed that the higher fertility when ewes were joined at 25 ewes per ram was associated with a faster rate of lamb drop during the first 4 weeks of lambing.

IV. DISCUSSION

With individual ram matings (experiments 1 and 3) a significantly lower proportion of ewes was mated during the first 14 days of joining in those treatments with a high number of ewes joined per ram. Even after 6 weeks of joining a greater proportion of ewes remained unmated in these treatments. Hafez (1951) has reported that ewes with a high level of sex drive actively seek out rams, an observation confirmed by Inkster (1957). Such ewes may compete for the favours of the ram to the successful exclusion of ewes of more passive or subservient behaviour (Lindsay and Robinson 1961a, 1961b; Banks 1964), and Lindsay and Robinson (1961a) found that the proportion of ewes escaping service in this way increased as the ratio of oestrous ewes to rams increased, in agreement with the results reported here.

With group ram matings (experiment 2), decreasing the number of ewes joined per ram was not associated with a higher proportion of ewes served in the first 14 days of joining. When rams are joined in groups, those of high libido are able to make up for their less active partners, thereby far exceeding the number of ewes they would mate if joined individually.

By increasing the number of ewes joined per ram, the actual number of ewes served per ram per day was markedly increased (Figs. 1(a), 2(a)). This probably led to a reduction in the number of services received by each oestrous ewe, as the occurrence of a lower frequency of service with increasing number of ewes in oestrus has been recorded previously for both pen (Hulet et al. 1962a, 1962c) and paddock (Mattner and Braden 1967; Mattner, Braden, and Turnbull 1967) matings. With group ram joinings there was, in addition, a reduction in the number of rams serving each oestrous ewe.

The most important result of this series of experiments was the increased flock fertility obtained by decreasing the number of ewes joined per ram. This result is at variance with that reported by Edgar (1965) in which no significant differences in fertility were obtained by flock matings at either one, two, or three rams per 100 ewes joined, and also contrasts with the conclusions drawn by Terrill and Stoehr (1939), Wiggins, Terrill, and Emik (1953) Haughey (1959), and Mattner and Braden (1967). The latter workers, however, noted a higher proportion of pregnancies in ewes served thrice or more than in those served once only, and there are several reports of increased ewe conception following two *v.* one insemination (Lysov and Stojanovskaja 1937; Sinclair 1957; Salamon and Robinson 1962; Dunlop and Tallis 1964). Additional services *per se*, quite independent of the deposition of sperm in the vagina, may also increase fertility as seen in the practice of post-inseminal teasing (Restall 1961). Support for the results of experiments reported here is seen in the recent work of Schäfer and Matter (1966). They found that the ewe conception rate declined from 54 to 35% as the number of ewes served per ram per night increased from two to five respectively.

It is likely that part of the variability between reports on this topic is due to the different climatic and nutritional conditions under which the experiments were conducted. However, a more tangible variable, clearly demonstrated in the results reported here, is the age or sexual maturity of the rams used in such experiments.

Whereas significant increases in fertility were obtained by decreasing the number of ewes joined to $1\frac{1}{2}$-year-old rams, this was not so with older rams (experiment 4, Table 7). The large differences in fertility between treatments in experiments 1, 2, and 3 were therefore probably due in part to the use of $1\frac{1}{2}$-year-old rams. The literature concerned with the effect of ram age on fertility is conflicting. Reporting on a series of large field trials, Haughey (1959) observed that "shearling" rams were of lower fertility than older rams but unfortunately gives no data on the magnitude of the effect. Other workers have reported no correlation between ram age and fertility (Terrill and Stoehr 1939; Wiggins, Terrill, and Emik 1953; Parker and Bell 1966) and in one instance decreasing fertility was associated with increasing age of rams from 1 to 8 years (Schäfer and Matter 1966).

Experiment 4 clearly demonstrated that older rams can give higher levels of flock fertility but that the effect depends, among other things, on the number of ewes joined per ram. Older rams were more fertile than the $1\frac{1}{2}$-year-old rams when joined at 50 ewes per ram but not when the ratio was reduced to 25 ewes per ram (interaction, $P < 0.001$). Even at the lower ratio, however, the older rams produced a quicker rate of lamb drop, 142 lambs being born 14 days after the start of mating compared with 88 by the younger rams (Fig. 4; $\chi_1^2 = 16.84$; $P < 0.001$).

The fertility response (13% lambs born, Table 8), obtained by decreasing the number of ewes joined per ram in experiment 5 with "mixed age" rams, contrasts with the lack of response with $2\frac{1}{2}$–$5\frac{1}{2}$-year-old rams only in experiment 4 (Table 7, experiments 4 and 5 are directly comparable). Part of this difference would be due to the lower fertility of the $1\frac{1}{2}$-year-old rams included in the mixed age ram groups. In addition, it is possible that the mating activity of the younger rams was restricted by dominant older rams (Hulet *et al.* 1962b), the effective ratio of ewes per ram being thereby increased.

173

A comparison of individual *v*. group ram matings in relation to the number of ewes joined per ram warrants consideration. It is reasonable to expect that fertility differences between any treatments involving group matings would be less than that observed with individual ram matings. In the latter instance rams of high fertility "settle" most of their allocated number of ewes during the first 17 days of joining, and so have few ewes to serve during the remaining 3–6 week period. When group-mated, fertile rams mate and "settle" additional ewes during the latter part of the joining period, as they have access to ewes returning to service by their less fertile partners. This situation is seen in the percentage of ewes lambing to individual *v*. group ram matings in the experiments described here (experiment 1, Table 2,

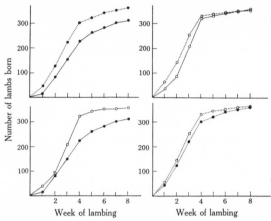

Fig. 4.—Interaction between number of ewes joined per ram and ram age on the cumulative number of lambs born each week: experiment 4. ● 1 ram/50 ewes. ○ 1/25. —— 1½-year-old rams. ····· 3½–5½-year-old rams.

Individual matings *v*. experiment 2, Table 4, Group matings). The difference between the two systems, individual *v*. group ram matings, is greatest when the ewe/ram ratio is high, as in this case variation in fertility between individual rams is at a maximum. For instance, in experiment 3 the range in fertility between individual rams was 46, 34, and 4% of ewes lambing for the 100, 50, and 25 ewes joined per ram treatments respectively (Table 5).

A further point to be considered is the period for which the rams are joined with the ewe flock. It can be generalized that as the period of mating is increased less difference is likely to be found between any two treatments comparing different numbers of ewes joined per ram. Experiment 4 provides an example where 3½–5½-year-old rams joined at 25 ewes per ram produced significantly more lambs than the young rams during the first 2 weeks of lambing (Fig. 4, 142 *v*. 88; $P < 0.001$) but no difference could be found between the two treatments at the conclusion of 8 weeks' lambing. Once again from experiment 4, 1½-year-old rams joined at 25 ewes per ram produced 95 more lambs during the first 4 weeks of lambing than those joined at 50 ewes per ram. At the conclusion of 8 weeks' lambing, however, this margin was reduced to 44 lambs, and it is likely that had the mating period been extended to 12 weeks the difference between treatments would have been reduced to a non-significant level.

The ewes in experiments 1 to 3 of this series had grazed pastures containing subterranean clover (*Trifolium subterraneum* L.) of the Dwalganup variety for periods of 3 to 5 years. This clover is oestrogenic (Davies and Bennett 1962; Beck 1964) and can produce infertility in ewes characterized by a reduced ability to conceive and abnormally high incidences of maternal dystocia, lamb mortality, and uterine prolapse (Bennetts, Underwood, and Shier 1946). Whereas these ewes had shown none of the more spectacular symptoms mentioned and their fertility in preceding years had been what is commonly accepted as "normal" (60–80% lambs marked) it is likely that their fertility was impaired to some extent as a result of oestrogenic grazing. Infertility following prolonged grazing on Dwalganup subterranean clover has recently been reported by Davenport (1967) and was subsequently shown by Lightfoot, Croker, and Neil (1967) to be associated with a failure of sperm transport through the ewe's genital tract. Impaired sperm transport also accompanies ewe infertility following prolonged grazing on red clover (Turnbull, Braden, and George 1966). In view of these facts it is possible that ewes of reduced fertility due to oestrogenic grazing are more responsive to increased number of services per ewe (Turnbull, Braden, and George 1966) such as would occur by joining fewer ewes per ram. Although the experiments reported here provide no direct comparison with normal ewes, a very large response (21% lambs born to ewes mated) was obtained with ewes of known infertility due to clover disease by reducing the number of ewes joined per ram in experiment 6 (Table 8).

Because there are many factors that can influence the relationship between number of ewes joined per ram and flock fertility, extensive extrapolation from these results to other environments may be unwise. The results do indicate, however, that field experimentation, particularly with reference to young rams, is warranted.

V. Acknowledgments

The authors wish to thank Mr. B. Vickers and Mr. M. White for their valuable assistance during the conduct of experiments 1, 2 and 3, and are indebted to Messrs. V. D. Cahill and Co., Nangeenan, on whose property experiments 4 and 5 were conducted. We would also like to thank Mr. H. G. Neil, Dr. H. Lloyd Davies, and Dr. M. Somers for their advice and encouragement. This project received financial support from the Australian Wool Board, to whom grateful acknowledgment is made.

VI. References

BANKS, E. M. (1964).—Some aspects of sexual behaviour in domestic sheep, *Ovis aries*. *Behaviour* **23**, 249–79.

BECK, A. B. (1964).—The oestrogenic isoflavones of subterranean clover. *Aust. J. agric. Res.* **15**, 223–30.

BENNETTS, H. W., UNDERWOOD, E. J., and SHIER, F. L. (1946).—A specific breeding problem of sheep on subterranean clover pastures in Western Australia. *Aust. vet. J.* **22**, 2–12.

BIGGERS, J. D. (1951).—The calculation of the dose-response line in quantal assays with special reference to oestrogen assays by the Allen-Doisy technique. *J. Endocr.* **8**, 169–78.

CLARINGBOLD, P. J., and EMMENS, C. W. (1961).—Quantal responses. *In* "Quantitative Methods in Pharmacology". (Ed. H. De Jonge.) pp. 72–87. (North Holland Publ. Co.: Amsterdam.)

DAVENPORT, N. (1967).—A measure of clover infertility in ewes. *J. Dep. Agric. West. Aust.* **8**, 83–8.

DAVIES, H. LLOYD, and BENNETT, D. (1962).—Studies on the oestrogenic activity of subterranean clover (*Trifolium subterraneum* L.) in south-western Australia. *Aust. J. agric. Res.* **13**, 1030–40.

DUNLOP, A. A., and TALLIS, G. M. (1964).—The effects of length of oestrus and number of inseminations on the fertility and twinning rate of the Merino ewe. *Aust. J. agric. Res.* **15**, 282–8.

EDGAR, D. G. (1965).—Talking about tupping. Proc. Ruakura Fmrs' Conf. Week, p. 61.

GREEN, W. W. (1947).—The duration of sperm fertility in the ewe. *Am. J. vet. Res.* **8**, 299–300.

HAFEZ, E. S. E. (1951).—Mating behaviour in sheep. *Nature, Lond.* **167**, 777.

HAUGHEY, K. G. (1959).—Preliminary report on a tupping survey. Sheepfmg A., pp. 17–26.

HULET, C. V., ERCANBRACK, S. K., PRICE, D. A., BLACKWELL, R. L., and WILSON, L. O. (1962*a*).— Mating behaviour of the ram in the one-sire pen. *J. Anim. Sci.* **21**, 857–64.

HULET, C. V., ERCANBRACK, S. K., BLACKWELL, R. L., PRICE, D. A., and WILSON, L. O. (1962*b*).— Mating behaviour of the ram in the multi-sire pen. *J. Anim. Sci.* **21**, 865–9.

HULET, C. V., BLACKWELL, R. L., ERCANBRACK, S. K., PRICE, D. A., and WILSON, L. O. (1962*c*).— Mating behaviour of the ewe. *J. Anim. Sci.* **21**, 870–4.

INKSTER, I. J. (1957).—The mating behaviour of sheep. Sheepfmg A., pp. 163–9.

LIGHTFOOT, R. J. (1968).—Studies on the number of ewes joined per ram for flock matings under paddock conditions. II. The effect of mating on semen characteristics. *Aust. J.agric.Res.* **19**, 1043–57.

LIGHTFOOT, R. J., CROKER, K. P., and NEIL, H. G. (1967).—Failure of sperm transport in relation to ewe infertility following prolonged grazing on oestrogenic pastures. *Aust. J. agric. Res.* **18**, 755–65.

LINDSAY, D. R., and ROBINSON, T. J. (1961*a*).—Studies on the efficiency of mating in the sheep. I. The effect of paddock size and number of rams. *J. agric. Sci., Camb.* **57**, 137–40.

LINDSAY, D. R., and ROBINSON, T. J. (1961*b*).—Studies on the efficiency of mating in the sheep. II. The effect of freedom of rams, paddock size and age of ewes. *J. agric. Sci., Camb.* **57**, 141–5.

LYSOV, A. M., and STOJANOVSKAJA, V. I. (1937).—[Increase in fertility of Karakal sheep.] *Problemy Zhivot.* **6**(12), 16.

MATTNER, P. E., and BRADEN, A. W. H. (1967).—Studies in flock mating of sheep. II. Fertilisation and prenatal mortality. *Aust. J. exp. Agric. Anim. Husb.* **7**, 110–16.

MATTNER, P. E., BRADEN, A. W. H., and TURNBULL, K. E. (1967).—Studies in flock mating of sheep. I. Mating behaviour. *Aust. J. exp. Agric. Anim. Husb.* **7**, 103–9.

PARKER, C. F., and BELL, D. S. (1966).—Factors associated with the ram influence on ewe fertility. Res. Summ. Ohio agric. Res. Devel. Center, No. 11, 1–5.

QUINLAN, J., MARÉ, G. S., and ROUX, L. L. (1933).—A study of the duration of motility of spermatozoa in the different divisions of the reproductive tract of the Merino ewe. *Onderstepoort J. vet. Sci. Anim. Ind.* **1**, 135–45.

RADFORD, H. M., WATSON, R. H., and WOOD, G. F. (1960).—A crayon and associated harness for the detection of mating under field conditions. *Aust. vet. J.* **36**, 57–66.

RESTALL, B. J. (1961).—Artificial insemination in sheep. VI. The effect of post-inseminal coitus on percentage of ewes lambing to a single insemination. *Aust. vet. J.* **37**, 70–2.

SALAMON, S., and ROBINSON, T. J. (1962).—Studies on the artificial insemination of Merino sheep. I. The effects of frequency and season of insemination, age of ewe, rams, and milk diluents on lambing performance. *Aust. J. agric. Res.* **13**, 52–68.

SCHÄFER, H., and MATTER, H. E. (1966).—Sexual behaviour of the ram in harem-mating, in relation to conception rate. *Züchtungskunde* **38**, 186–92.

SINCLAIR, A. N. (1957).—The effect of variation of mating, mating frequency and semen dose rate on conception in Merino sheep. *Aust. vet. J.* **33**, 88–91.

STARKE, N. C. (1949).—The sperm picture of rams of different breeds as an indication of their fertility. II. The rate of sperm travel in the genital tract of the ewe. *Onderstepoort J. vet. Sci. Anim. Ind.* **22**, 415–525.

TERRILL, C. E., and STOEHR, J. A. (1939).—Reproduction in range sheep. *Rec. Proc. Am. Soc. Anim. Prod.* **32**, 369–75.

TURNBULL, K. E., BRADEN, A. W. H., and GEORGE, J. M. (1966).—Fertilization and early embryonic losses in ewes that had grazed oestrogenic pastures for 6 years. *Aust. J. agric. Res.*, **17**, 907–17.

WIGGINS, E. L., TERRILL, C. E., and EMIK, L. O. (1953).—Relationships between libido semen characteristics and fertility in range rams. *J. Anim. Sci.* **12**, 684–96.

STUDIES ON THE NUMBER OF EWES JOINED PER RAM FOR FLOCK MATINGS UNDER PADDOCK CONDITIONS

II. THE EFFECT OF MATING ON SEMEN CHARACTERISTICS

By R. J. Lightfoot

I. Introduction

In the study of flock infertility when ewes are mated by unrestrained rams in large paddocks, it is frequently difficult to identify reproductive failure due to the ram, as opposed to that of female origin. Investigation of the ram requires data on the nature and significance of the seminal changes that occur during paddock joinings. Although there are many reports in the literature concerned with ram semen characteristics, the majority of these deal with rams subjected to low rates of ejaculation. If oestrous ewes are readily available, the unrestrained ram will complete many services each day (Hulet *et al.* 1962a, 1962b; Mattner, Braden, and Turnbull 1967) and it is known that frequent ejaculation results in rapid diminution in ejaculate volume, sperm density, and their product, total number of sperm per ejaculate (Salamon 1962, 1964).

Gunn, Saunders, and Granger (1942) have made observations on ram semen prior to and during mating and found depletion of sperm numbers during the joining period, and recently Mattner and Braden (1967) have described a rapid fall in ejaculate sperm numbers coincident with the onset of mating.

The experiments reported here provide information on the effect of mating on some semen characteristics, particularly in relation to the number of ewes joined per ram.

TABLE 1

PRINCIPAL FEATURES OF DESIGN AND CONDUCT FOR ALL EXPERIMENTS

Experiment No.:	1	2	3
Design	Factorial (2×3)	Single classification	Factorial (4×4)
Treatments	Rams/ewes:	Rams ($1\frac{1}{2}$ years old)/ewes:	Rams/ewes:
	(1)† 1/100 (300)‡	(1) 1/100 (300)	(1) 1/100 (400)
	(2)† 1/40 (120)	(2) 1/40 (120)	(2) 1/50 (200)
			(3) 1/25 (100)
			(4) Unmated rams (0)
	Ram liveweight:	Rams ($2\frac{1}{2}$ years old)/ewes:	Sperm/ejaculate:
	Low (140)	(3) 1/40 (120)	$4\cdot0 \times 10^9$ (175)
	Medium (140)	(4) Unmated	$3\cdot4 \times 10^9$ (175)
	High (140)	rams (0)	$2\cdot8 \times 10^9$ (175)
			$2\cdot2 \times 10^9$ (175)
Total no. of rams	6	12	16
Total no. of ewes	420	540	700
Age of rams	$1\frac{1}{2}$ years	$1\frac{1}{2}$ v. $2\frac{1}{2}$ years	$1\frac{1}{2}$ years
Age of ewes	3–6 years	3–6 years	2–6 years
Ram joining	Individual	Group	Individual
Date of joining	14.ii.1963	18.ii.1964	3.iii.1965
Period of joining	6 weeks	6 weeks	6 weeks
Method of semen collection	Electroejaculation	Electroejaculation	Artificial vagina

† Treatment No. referred to in text.　　‡ Number of ewes per treatment given in parenthesis.

II. Materials and Methods

Details of the animals used and the conditions under which they were joined are given by Lightfoot and Smith (1968). The principal features of design and conduct for the three experiments concerned with semen collection are shown in Table 1. Methods used for semen collection and evaluation are given below.

(a) Experiment 1

Semen was collected by the electroejaculation technique (Blackshaw 1954) at weekly intervals commencing 3 weeks prior to and continuing throughout the joining

178

period. Ejaculate volume was measured and visual assessments of ejaculate consistency, wave motion (score 0 to 5), and percentage motile sperm (nearest 20%) recorded. Consistency classifications were expressed as approximate sperm density equivalents according to the conversion suggested by Mattner and Moule (1965). This conversion is similar to that reported by Gunn, Saunders, and Granger (1942).

Consistency classification:	Thick creamy	Creamy	Thin creamy	Milky	Cloudy	Almost clear
Approx. sperm density ($10^{-9} \times$ No. of sperm/ml):	4·0	3·0	2·0	1·0	0·5	0·1

A portion of each ejaculate was stained with nigrosin-eosin (Hancock 1952) and slides prepared for observations on sperm morphology. These were scored either 3, 2, or 1, representing approximately less than 10%, 10–20%, and more than 20% morphologically abnormal sperm respectively.

(b) Experiment 2

On one occasion prior to, twice during, and once 2 days after the conclusion of joining an ejaculate was collected from each ram (electroejaculation) and examined as described for experiment 1. The three unmated rams (treatment 4) were run under paddock conditions and semen was tested on the same days as those joined with ewes (treatments 1–3).

(c) Experiment 3

On four occasions prior to and at intervals of 4 days throughout the joining period ejaculates were collected from each of the 16 rams by artificial vagina (Anderson 1945; Salamon and Lindsay 1961). Ejaculate volume was measured, wave motion scored (0–5), and sperm density determined by the photoelectric absorptiometer method (Comstock and Green 1939). Reaction time, defined as the interval from the rams' initial approach to ejaculation, was recorded. Semen smears stained with nigrosin-eosin were examined for percentage unstained sperm (Campbell, Dott, and Glover 1956) and percentage morphologically abnormal sperm (Hancock 1952).

(d) Statistical Analyses

The effects of treatments on semen characteristics in the three experiments were tested by analysis of variance. Day of collection was examined as a split plot factor and its significance tested against the appropriate error mean square (Snedecor 1956).

In experiment 3, simple correlation coefficients between semen characteristics were calculated for both mating (rams in treatments 1, 2, and 3 during joining; 108 observations) and non-mating rams (rams in all treatments prior to and after joining plus treatment 4 rams throughout joining; 72 observations). The correlation coefficients calculated on a within-treatment basis were not different so only those calculated for the pooled data from all treatments are presented.

179

As semen was collected from all mating rams every 4 days throughout joining, both the number of ewes served and ewe conception rate (ewes lambing/ewes served) during the series of 4 day periods, commencing either 4, 3, 2, 1, or 0 days prior to each collection, were tested for correlation with the semen characteristics observed on that collection day.

III. Results

(a) Experiment 1

(i) Ejaculate Volume, Sperm Density, and Total Number of Sperm per Ejaculate

Ejaculate volume and sperm density fell markedly after the onset of mating (Table 2), the effect being shown statistically by a highly significant effect for day of collection (volume, $P < 0.01$; density, $P < 0.001$). There were, however, no significant

TABLE 2

SEMEN CHARACTERISTICS PRIOR TO AND DURING JOINING: EXPERIMENT 1 (TREATMENT MEANS)

Day of Semen Collection (1963)	Ejaculate Volume (ml)		$10^{-9} \times$ Sperm Density (No. of sperm/ml)		Wave Motion Score (0–5)	
	Rams/ewes: 1/100	1/40	1/100	1/40	1/100	1/40
Jan. 31	1·1	0·6	2·33	1·67	1·67	1·67
Feb. 7	1·9	1·1	1·33	2·00	2·00	1·67
Feb. 14	1·1	1·0	2·33	3·00	3·00	3·00
Mean (pre-joining)	1·4	0·9	2·00	2·22	2·22	2·11
Feb. 21	0·8	0·6	0·37	0·83	0·33	0·33
Feb. 28	0·9	0·5	0·37	0·67	0·33	0·33
Mar. 7	0·6	0·6	0·23	0·30	0·00	0·00
Mar. 14	0·6	0·5	1·20	1·33	0·67	1·00
Mar. 21	0·4	0·6	1·20	1·20	0·33	0·33
Mar. 28	0·3	0·8	0·67	1·33	0·33	1·67
Mean (during joining)	0·6	0·6	0·67	0·94	0·33	0·61

differences between rams joined to either 100 or 40 ewes. "Medium" liveweight rams produced ejaculates of greater sperm density than rams of either "Low" or "High" liveweight ($P < 0.001$), but there was evidence of an interaction ($P < 0.05$) between ram liveweight group and day of collection.

Total number of sperm per ejaculate dropped markedly after the beginning of mating (Fig. 1), the effect being shown by a highly significant ($P < 0.001$) collection day effect. There was no significant difference between the treatments, although there were indications that treatment 2 (one ram/40 ewes) showed better recovery than treatment 1 (one ram/100 ewes) towards the end of joining. There was heterogeneity ($P < 0.01$) between the three ram liveweight groups, Low rams yielding con-

180

siderably fewer total sperm per ejaculate than either Medium or High rams (0·48 v. 1·51 and 1·36 × 10⁹ sperm respectively).

(ii) *Wave Motion and Sperm Morphology*

Wave motion score decreased markedly during the joining period (Table 2; $P < 0·01$), the effect being due to a fall in sperm density rather than reduced velocity of the individual sperm cells. There was an effect of ram group (Medium > Low and High; $P < 0·01$) but no difference between the two main treatments.

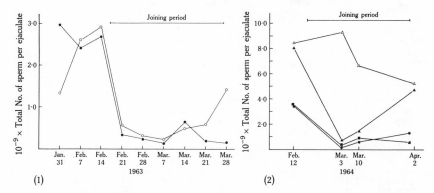

Figs. 1 and 2.—Effect of mating on ram semen characteristics: total number of sperm per ejaculate.

Fig. 1.—Experiment 1. Treatments: ● (1) 1 ram/100 ewes; (○) (2) 1 ram/40 ewes.

Fig. 2.—Experiment 2. Treatments: ■ (1) 3 1½-year-old rams/300 ewes; ● (2) 3 1½-year-old rams/120 ewes; ▲ (3) 3 2½-year-old rams/120 ewes; △ (4) 3 unmated rams.

The percentage of motile sperm in the ejaculate showed similar trends to wave motion score, but the ram group and collection day effects just failed to achieve statistical significance ($0·05 < P < 0·1$).

Semen smears obtained prior to joining were interesting in that most rams showed evidence of seminal degeneration ($> 10\%$ morphologically abnormal sperm) on one of the first, second, or third collection days. Only one of the six rams showed less than 10% abnormal cells on all three occasions. During joining, observations on sperm morphology could not be obtained in six instances owing to insufficient sperm being present on the smear. The morphology scores (maximum 3) for treatment 1 were 2·2 v. 2·4 for prior to and during the joining period respectively, and 2·8 v. 2·5 in the case of treatment 2. Chi-square analysis of these scores revealed no significant effects. Detached heads or coiled and bent tails comprised the majority of the morphological abnormalities observed.

(b) *Experiment 2*

Trends in ejaculate volume and sperm density (Table 3) and their product, total number of sperm per ejaculate (Fig. 2), were similar within each treatment. There were significant differences between treatments (ejaculate volume and sperm density, $P < 0.01$; total number of sperm per ejaculate, $P < 0.001$), although several effects contributed to this variance component. Young rams (treatments 1 and 2) were markedly lower than the older rams (treatments 3 and 4) at the collections

TABLE 3

SEMEN CHARACTERISTICS PRIOR TO, DURING, AND AFTER JOINING: EXPERIMENT 2 (TREATMENT MEANS)

Joining period: Feb. 18 to Mar. 31, 1964
Treatment 1: three 1½-year-old rams/300 ewes
Treatment 2: three 1½-year-old rams/120 ewes
Treatment 3: three 2½-year-old rams/120 ewes
Treatment 4: three 2½-year-old rams not mated (control)

Day of Semen Collection (1964)	Ejaculate Volume (ml)				$10^{-9} \times$ Sperm Density (No. of sperm/ml)				Wave Motion Score (0–5)			
Treatment:	1	2	3	4	1	2	3	4	1	2	3	4
Feb. 12	1·5	1·4	2·7	2·2	3·3	3·3	4·0	4·7	2·0	1·3	1·3	1·7
Mar. 3	0·6	0·8	0·8	2·3	1·0	0·3	1·3	5·0	0·3	0·0	1·3	4·7
Mar. 10	0·8	0·4	0·7	1·8	2·0	1·7	2·3	4·7	1·7	1·7	2·7	3·7
Apr. 2	0·6	0·9	1·4	1·7	2·3	2·3	4·0	4·0	0·7	1·3	0·7	3·7
Means	0·88	0·88	1·40	2·00	2·15	1·90	2·90	4·60	1·18	1·08	1·50	3·45

prior to and at the conclusion of joining (Fig. 2). In addition, with treatments 1, 2, and 3, large falls in all semen characteristics occurred on the two collection days during joining, contrasting with high values maintained by the control (unmated) rams (treatment 4).

TABLE 4

SEMEN CHARACTERISTICS PRIOR TO AND DURING JOINING:
EXPERIMENT 3: SUMMARY OF ANALYSIS OF VARIANCE
All figures are variance ratios other than error mean squares shown in italics

Effect	Degrees of Freedom	Ejaculate Volume	Sperm Density	Sperm Density† (d.f.)	Total No. of Sperm per Ejaculate
Treatment (A)	3	23·04***	2·88	6·17*	19·38***
Ram group (B)	3	0·82	0·88	1·48	0·77
A × B (error 1)	9	*0·132*	*304·0*	*135·6*	*237·1*
Collection day (C)	15	7·61***	11·26***	5·92**(3)	11·37***
A × C	45	2·89***	1·18	1·10 (9)	2·66***
B × C	45	1·25	0·76	0·58 (9)	1·23
A × B × C (error 2)	135	*0·052*	*44·6*	*36·2* (27)	*78·28*

* $P < 0.05$.   ** $P < 0.01$.   *** $P < 0.001$

† Data from the first four collection days after the start of joining only (Mar. 11, 15, 19, and 23). Figures in parenthesis refer to the degrees of freedom for the effects of collection day and its interactions.

There were significant differences between collection days (ejaculate volume and total number of sperm per ejaculate, $P < 0.05$; sperm density, $P < 0.01$).

The unmated rams yielded high mean values for both wave motion score (Table 3) and percentage motile sperm, but there were no differences between treatments 1–3 nor between collection days.

(c) Experiment 3

(i) Ejaculate Volume

There was a highly significant difference between treatments ($P < 0.001$) due to the control rams (treatment 4) maintaining ejaculate volume throughout the experi-

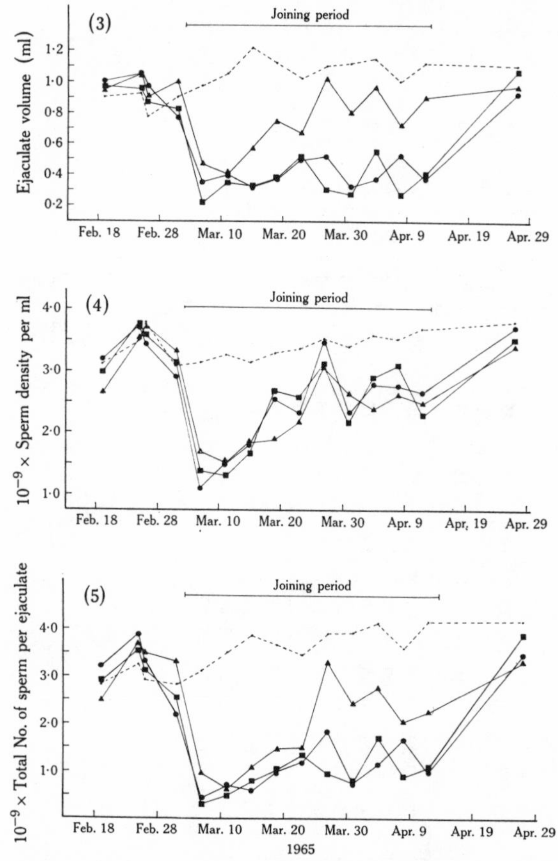

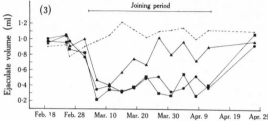

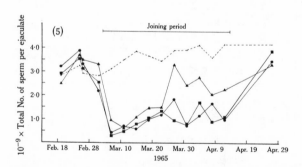

Figs. 3–5.—Effect of mating on ram semen characteristics, experiment 3.

Fig. 3.—Ejaculate volume.

Fig. 4.—Sperm density.

Fig. 5.—Total No. of sperm per ejaculate.

Treatments:
● (1) 1 ram/100 ewes.
■ (2) 1 ram/50 ewes.
▲ (3) 1 ram/25 ewes.
--- (4) Control, not mated.

ment (Fig. 3). A highly significant effect was also obtained for day of collection ($P < 0.001$; Table 4) even though the control rams showed little variation compared with the characteristic drop in ejaculate volume at the start of the joining period in treatments 1, 2, and 3. The highly significant ($P < 0.001$) treatment × collection day interaction is due in part to this result, but also is a result of the comparatively early recovery in ejaculate volume by treatment 3 rams (one ram/25 ewes).

Table 5

SEMEN CHARACTERISTICS PRIOR TO AND DURING JOINING: EXPERIMENT 3 (TREATMENT MEANS)

Treatment 1: 1 ram/100 ewes; treatment 2: 1 ram/50 ewes; treatment 3: 1 ram/25 ewes; treatment 4: control, unmated

Day of Semen Collection (1965)	Wave Motion Score (0–5)				Stained Sperm (%)				Morph. Abnormal Sperm (%)				Reaction Time (sec)			
Treatment:	1	2	3	4	1	2	3	4	1	2	3	4	1	2	3	4
Feb. 25	4·25	4·75	4·50	5·00					1·9	2·6	3·4	1·8	43	116	46	64
Feb. 26	4·50	4·75	2·75	4·75					2·8	6·1	2·5	1·6	53	93	78	61
Mar. 3	4·25	3·50	2·00	4·75	34	34	47	24					41	96	112	83
Means (pre-joining)	4·33	4·33	3·08	4·83	34	34	47	24	2·4	4·4	2·9	1·7	46	102	79	69
Mar. 7	3·50	3·50	3·75	4·25	26	38	30	20	2·2	10·9	2·4	1·1	80	201	171	231
Mar. 11	2·50	3·00	3·00	4·25	14	15	30	8	4·9	2·7	1·3	0·8	230	349	52	84
Mar. 15	3·00	2·75	3·00	4·50	16	23	12	12	4·4	9·4	10·3	3·6	97	285	158	58
Mar. 19	4·75	4·75	4·75	4·75	14	21	15	10	18·3	19·7	5·9	1·8	314	423	407	92
Mar. 23	4·50	5·00	3·75	4·25	8	4	14	11	4·4	4·5	1·3	1·3	147	294	129	82
Mar. 27	4·75	4·75	4·75	3·75	8	9	21	18	2·1	3·7	3·8	3·2	172	310	158	163
Mar. 31	3·75	3·75	4·75	4·75	5	11	6	9	1·5	4·3	1·3	2·6	86	253	190	95
Apr. 4	4·00	3·00	3·25	4·25	12	27	34	14	2·0	2·7	2·3	3·7	310	306	301	89
Apr. 8	3·00	3·25	4·25	4·25	30	27	17	7	3·9	3·3	2·8	1·6	536	255	264	99
Apr. 12	4·25	3·00	3·25	3·50	21	35	31	19	1·6	8·4	5·3	2·6	374	309	377	172
Means (during joining)	3·80	3·68	3·75	4·25	15·4	21·0	21·0	12·8	4·53	6·96	3·67	2·23	235	299	221	117
Apr. 27	4·75	4·75	4·00	4·75	13	16	16	8	2·1	2·7	2·3	3·4	125	186	109	80
Overall means	3·98	3·89	3·63	4·41	16·8	21·7	22·8	13·3	4·01	6·23	3·45	2·24	186	248	182	104

184

(ii) *Sperm Density*

The only significant effect on sperm density was that of collection day (Table 4; $P < 0.001$). In contrast to results of ejaculate volume, there was no significant treatment effect nor a treatment $\times$ collection day interaction, although treatment means show these trends in Figure 4. By analysing the data for the first 4 collection days after the start of joining only, the treatment effect can be demonstrated statistically ($P < 0.05$; Table 4).

Sperm density also differed from ejaculate volume in that all "mating" treatments showed progressive recovery to a similar extent after the initial fall at the start of joining. Treatment 3 was not superior.

(iii) *Total Number of Sperm per Ejaculate*

Although total sperm per ejaculate is influenced by both ejaculate volume and sperm density, statistically significant effects followed those of ejaculate volume rather than the latter semen characteristic (Table 4). Highly significant effects ($P < 0.001$) were obtained for treatments, days of collection, and their interaction. As with ejaculate volume, the treatment $\times$ collection day interaction is a result both of the sudden fall in total sperm shown by treatments 1 to 3 at the start of mating, and also of the greater relative recovery of treatment 3 towards the middle of the joining period (Fig. 5). There were no significant differences between treatments 1, 2, and 3 during the first 16 days of joining.

(iv) *Wave Motion Score and Ram Reaction Time*

There was significant ($P < 0.001$) variation between collection days, the main effect being a slight depression in wave motion score early in the joining period (Table 5). This results contrasts with the marked depression in wave motion score that occurred during joining in experiment 1, and is probably explained by the much lower sperm density of ejaculates obtained by electroejaculation in that experiment.

Reaction time also varied significantly between collection days ($P < 0.001$), there being a marked increase at the beginning of joining. The effect, however, was modified by interactions with both treatment and ram groups. The treatment $\times$ collection day interaction was mainly due to the increase in reaction time during joining in treatments 1–3 (Table 5).

(v) *Percentage Stained Sperm*

There was marked variation in percentage stained ("dead") sperm both within treatments and within rams between collection days. A significant effect of collection day ($P < 0.001$) was found but this did not seem to be affected by either treatment (Table 5) or ram group.

Total unstained sperm per ejaculate followed essentially similar trends to those seen in total sperm per ejaculate except that the treatment $\times$ collection day interaction was not as large ($P < 0.05$ *v.* $P < 0.001$).

(vi) *Percentage Abnormal Sperm*

The incidence of morphologically abnormal sperm in the ejaculate was statistically unrelated to either treatment or ram group but varied markedly between collection days ($P < 0.001$). The percentage of abnormal sperm reached a peak during the period 12–16 days after the start of joining (Table 5). Five of the 12 rams allocated to the mating treatments (treatments 1, 2, and 3) produced ejaculates containing more than 10% abnormal sperm on at least one collection day (Fig. 6). The most common

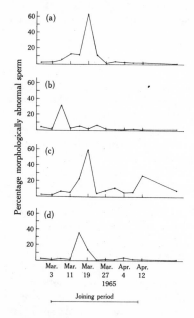

Fig. 6.—Incidence of morphologically abnormal sperm in the ejaculate of individual rams during joining, experiment 3.

(*a*) Treatment 1, ram 1.
    Peak: 40% DH, 10% CT, 50% P.

(*b*) Treatment 2, ram 2.
    Peak: 40% DH, 40% CT, 20% BT.

(*c*) Treatment 2, ram 4.
    First peak: 50% DH, 10% CT, 20% BT, 20% P.
    Second peak: 40% DH, 40% CT, 20% BT.

(*d*) Treatment 3, ram 2.
    Peak: 100% BT.

DH, detached head.

CT, coiled tail.

BT, bent tail.

P, pyriform head.

abnormalities were detached heads, coiled and bent tails, and to a lesser extent pyriform heads. In nearly all cases the elevated level occurred on one day only and was not evident on collection days immediately preceding or following the rise.

Total normal sperm per ejaculate showed similar trends and levels of significance to those obtained for total number of sperm per ejaculate.

(vii) *Simple Correlation Coefficients*

Simple correlation coefficients between all semen characteristics and other relevant parameters for both mating and non-mating rams are presented in Table 6.

Whereas wave motion score was positively and significantly related to ejaculate volume, sperm density, and total number of sperm per ejaculate in the case of mating rams, the relative coefficients were all low and non-significant for non-mating rams. This result is probably a reflection of the fact that the dense ejaculates of the non-mating rams almost invariably received the maximum score. Wave motion score was negatively correlated with percentage stained sperm in both mating and non-mating rams.

The number of ewes served during the 4 day period preceding semen collections was significantly and negatively correlated with total number of sperm per ejaculate (Fig. 7) and its two components, ejaculate volume and sperm density.

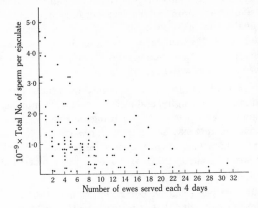

Fig. 7.—Relationship between the number of ewes served during the 4 days prior to semen collection and the total number of sperm obtained per ejaculate.

$r = -0.48***$.

The percentage of ewes lambing as a result of service during the 4 day period commencing 3 days prior to each semen collection was weakly — but surprisingly,

TABLE 6

CORRELATION COEFFICIENTS BETWEEN SEMEN CHARACTERISTICS AND OTHER ASPECTS OF REPRODUCTIVE PERFORMANCE: EXPERIMENT 3

Upright numerals, mating rams; italic numerals, non-mating rams

Observation	Sperm Density	Total No. Sperm per Ejaculate	Wave Motion Score	Reaction Time	Stained Sperm (%)	Abnormal Sperm (%)	No. of Ewes Served	Ewes Lambing (%)
Ejaculate volume	0·37***	0·91***	0·27**	0·05	−0·00	−0·19	−0·43***	−0·24*
	0·20	*0·84***	*0·08*	*0·04*	*−0·18*	*−0·19*		
Sperm density		0·65***	0·57***	−0·02	−0·19*	−0·09	−0·39***	−0·22*
		*0·70***	*0·09*	*0·23**	*−0·20*	*0·04*		
Total number of sperm per ejaculate			0·37***	0·02	−0·03	−0·15	−0·48***	−0·34***
			0·11	*0·10*	*−0·25**	*−0·08*		
Wave motion score				0·09	−0·54***	−0·22*	−0·18	−0·01
				*0·24**	*−0·78***	*−0·20*		
Reaction time					−0·10	0·06	−0·11	−0·11
					−0·20	*−0·16*		
Percentage of stained sperm						0·36***	0·04	−0·02
						*0·29**		
Percentage of abnormal sperm							0·14	−0·00

* $P<0.05$.　　** $P<0.01$.　　*** $P<0.001$.

negatively — related to the semen characteristics observed at that collection. The only significant correlation coefficients were those related to total number of sperm per ejaculate.

187

IV. Discussion

Semen was collected by electroejaculation in experiments 1 and 2 but by artificial vagina in experiment 3. Electroejaculation results in ejaculates of greater volume, lower sperm concentration, and similar but more variable levels of total numbers of sperm per ejaculate than those obtained by artificial vagina (Mattner and Voglmayr 1962). The artificial vagina probably yields ejaculates which more closely resemble those deposited in the ewe's vagina during natural mating (Terrill 1940) and therefore is to be preferred for the study of semen characteristics during joining.

In all three experiments the onset of mating was accompanied by a sudden and pronounced drop in ejaculate volume, sperm density, and their product, total number of sperm per ejaculate. Gunn, Saunders, and Granger (1942), using the electroejaculation technique, reported that paddock mating may have a temporary adverse effect on spermatogenesis, and of the semen characters sperm numbers were most affected. Unfortunately, in much of their work, "mated" rams were 1 to 2 years older and received a higher level of nutrition than "unmated" animals.

The fall in total sperm numbers per ejaculate coincident with the onset of mating reported herein agrees very closely with that reported recently by Mattner and Braden (1967) from daily artificial vagina collections during paddock matings. It occurs during the first 1 or 2 days of mating and resembles that resulting from frequent ejaculation with the artificial vagina (Salamon 1962, 1964; Salamon and Lightfoot 1967). Equilibrium values of $c.$ $0 \cdot 2$–$0 \cdot 8 \times 10^9$ sperm per ejaculate are achieved soon after the initial fall. These treatment means are higher than the figure of approximately $0 \cdot 13 \times 10^9$ sperm (in an inseminate volume of $0 \cdot 1$ ml) found by Salamon (1962) to result in maximum fertility to artificial insemination. During joining in experiments 1, 2, and 3, 10 out of 36, 2 of 18, and 5 of 120 ejaculates collected respectively contained less than $0 \cdot 13 \times 10^9$ total sperm. It is probable, however, that an ejaculate containing considerably more than this number of sperm is required to obtain maximum fertility to a single natural service when semen is deposited in the anterior vagina rather than directly into the entrance of the cervical canal as with artificial insemination (Dun 1955; Sarapa 1967).

It is interesting to note that in experiment 3 the ejaculate volume remained at a low level ($0 \cdot 2$–$0 \cdot 5$ ml) in treatments 1 and 2 throughout the joining period, but sperm density showed progressive recovery after the first 4 days of joining (Figs. 3, 4). Early recovery of sperm density rather than ejaculate volume may have a beneficial effect on fertility, as experiments with artificial insemination have shown a good relationship between sperm density and subsequent fertility when a constant inseminate volume was used (Salamon 1962), but increasing inseminate volume above $0 \cdot 1$ ml does not usually improve fertility (Robinson 1956, 1958; Sinclair 1957). Similarly, Hulet and Ercanbrack (1962) obtained a correlation coefficient of $0 \cdot 56$ ($P < 0 \cdot 001$) between sperm density and ewe fertility to natural service, whereas the coefficient for ejaculate volume was low and non-significant.

It has been reported that the onset of paddock mating may be accompanied by seminal degeneration with a high incidence of morphologically abnormal sperm in the ejaculate, the effect being most severe in hot environments (Gunn, Saunders, and Granger 1942). In the present study the incidence of abnormalities was usually low but during joining individual rams showed occasional large increases in the proportion of both abnormal and stained sperm. The effect was seldom evident for more than one or two collections and resembled that seen in ejaculates from a proportion of the rams (type C) studied by Moule and Waites (1963). Such rams yielded only one or two ejaculates of inferior quality after exposure to a temperature of 105°F for two 6 hr periods. The rams studied by Fowler (1965) also showed a similar degree of seminal degeneration when semen-tested during the hot summer months of eastern Australia. High ambient temperatures experienced prior to and throughout the early part of joining each year were possibly the main factor responsible for the sporadic seminal degeneration observed in the present results. During the January–February period there were 11–12 days in each of the years 1963, 1964, and 1965 on which maximum temperatures of greater than 100°F were recorded.

A considerable difference in both ejaculate volume and sperm density was found between $1\frac{1}{2}$- and $2\frac{1}{2}$-year-old rams, both before and after joining in experiment 2. The older rams also gave superior ejaculates during the joining period and it is likely that their better semen quality was a factor contributing to the higher lambing percentage obtained in that treatment. A clear difference in the fertility of older over $1\frac{1}{2}$-year-old rams was subsequently demonstrated by Lightfoot and Smith (1968).

Highly significant and negative correlation coefficients were found for ejaculate volume, sperm density, and total sperm per ejaculate in each case with the number of ewes served during the 4 days preceding semen collection. This relationship, shown for total sperm per ejaculate in Figure 7, suggests the occurrence of a maximum value dependent on the number of ewes served and declining as the number of ewes served increased. The actual values observed varied below this figure, probably according to the number of services given to each ewe.

A surprising result in the present study was the negative correlation coefficients found between semen characteristics during paddock joining and ewe conception rate. This result contrasts with positive relationships reported by Terrill (1937), Wiggins, Terrill, and Emik (1953), Hulet and Ercanbrack (1962), and Hulet, Foote and Blackwell (1965). It is possible that during paddock joining, and in the absence of severe seminal degeneration, a ram's relative fertility is determined both by the number of times he serves each oestrous ewe and by the total number of ewes served, rather than the quality of the semen voided. The demonstration of a significant relationship between prejoining libido and subsequent fertility (Wiggins, Terrill, and Emik 1953) supports this hypothesis. Highly fertile rams would therefore give ejaculates containing comparatively low total sperm numbers during the joining period, as occurred in experiment 3 when rams were joined individually to flocks of 100 ewes.

Such an example highlights the need for further research on the relative contributions of behavioural and seminal characteristics to ram fertility during paddock joining.

V. Acknowledgments

The author wishes to thank Messrs. K. P. Croker, M. White, F. Wilkinson, and Dr. S. M. Dennis for their valuable assistance during the experiments; and Mr. H. G. Neil, Dr. H. Lloyd Davies, and Dr. M. Somers for their advice and encouragement. This project received financial support from the Australian Wool Board, to whom grateful acknowledgment is made.

VI. References

ANDERSON, J. (1945).—Artificial insemination: the semen of animals and its use for artificial insemination. Tech. Commun. imp. Bur. Anim. Breed. Genet. No. 6.

BLACKSHAW, A. W. (1954).—A bipolar rectal electrode for the electrical production of ejaculation in sheep. *Aust. vet. J.* **30**, 249–50.

CAMPBELL, R. C., DOTT, H. M., and GLOVER, T. D. (1956).—Nigrosin-eosin as a stain for differentiating live and dead spermatozoa. *J. agric. Sci., Camb.* **48**, 1–8.

COMSTOCK, R. E., and GREEN, W. W. (1939).—Methods for semen evaluation. I. Density, respiration, glycolysis of semen. *Rec. Proc. Am. Soc. Anim. Prod.* **32**, 213–16.

DUN, R. B. (1955).—Quoted by Morrant, A. J., and Dun, R. B. (1960).—Artificial insemination of sheep. II. Techniques and equipment used at Trangie Agricultural Experiment Station. *Aust. vet. J.* **36**, 1–6.

FOWLER, D. G. (1965).—Semen quality of Merino rams. I. The effects of fleece length and season on semen quality. *Aust. J. exp. Agric. Anim. Husb.* **5**, 243–6.

GUNN, R. M. C., SAUNDERS, R. N., and GRANGER, W. (1942).—Studies in fertility in sheep. 2. Seminal changes affecting fertility in rams. Bull. Coun. scient. ind. Res. Aust. No. 148.

HANCOCK, J. L. (1952).—The morphology of bull spermatozoa. *J. exp. Biol.* **29**, 445–53.

HULET, C. V., and ERCANBRACK, S. K. (1962).—A fertility index for rams. *J. Anim. Sci.* **21**, 489–93.

HULET, C. V., ERCANBRACK, S. K., PRICE, D. A., BLACKWELL, R. L., and WILSON, L. O. (1962a).—Mating behaviour of the ram in the one-sire pen. *J. Anim. Sci.* **21**, 857–64.

HULET, C. V., ERCANBRACK, S. K., BLACKWELL, R. L., PRICE, D. A., and WILSON, L. O. (1962b).—Mating behaviour of the ram in the multi-sire pen. *J. Anim. Sci.* **21**, 865–9.

HULET, C. V., FOOTE, W. C., and BLACKWELL, R. L. (1965).—Relationship between semen quality and fertility in the ram to fecundity in the ewe. *J. Reprod. Fert.* **9**, 311–15.

LIGHTFOOT, R. J., and SMITH, J. A. C. (1968).—Studies on the number of ewes joined per ram for flock matings under paddock conditions. I. Mating behaviour and fertility. *Aust. J. agric. Res.* **19**, 1029–42.

MATTNER, P. E., and BRADEN, A. W. H. (1967).—Studies in flock mating of sheep. 2. Fertilization and prenatal mortality. *Aust. J. exp. Agric. Anim. Husb.* **7**, 110–16.

MATTNER, P. E., BRADEN, A. W. H., and TURNBULL, K. E. (1967).—Studies in flock mating of sheep. 1. Mating behaviour. *Aust. J. exp. Agric. Anim. Husb.* **7**, 103–9.

MATTNER, P. E., and MOULE, G. R. (1965).—Field investigations with sheep — a manual of techniques. (Ed. G. R. Moule.) pp. 11–21. (CSIRO Aust.: Melbourne.)

MATTNER, P. E., and VOGLMAYR, J. K. (1962).—A comparison of ram semen collected by the artificial vagina and by electroejaculation. *Aust. J. exp. Agric. Anim. Husb.* **2**, 78–81.

MOULE, G. R., and WAITES, G. M. H. (1963).—Seminal degeneration in the ram and its relation to the temperature of the scrotum. *J. Reprod. Fert.* **5**, 433–46.

ROBINSON, T. J. (1956).—The artificial insemination of the Merino sheep following the synchronization of oestrus and ovulation by progesterone injected alone and with pregnant mare serum gonadotrophin (PMS). *Aust. J. agric. Res.* **7**, 194–210.

ROBINSON, T. J. (1958).—Studies in controlled artificial insemination of Merino sheep. *Aust. J. agric. Res.* **9**, 693–703.

SALAMON, S. (1962).—Studies on the artificial insemination of Merino sheep. III. The effect of frequent ejaculation on semen characteristics and fertilizing capacity. *Aust. J. agric. Res.* **13**, 1137–50.

SALAMON, S. (1964).—The effect of frequent ejaculation in the ram on some semen characteristics. *Aust. J. agric. Res.* **15**, 950–60.

SALAMON, S., and LIGHTFOOT, R. J. (1967).—Effect of cold shock, liquid storage, and pellet-freezing on successive ram ejaculates. *Aust. J. agric. Res.* **18**, 959–72.

SALAMON, S., and LINDSAY, D. R. (1961).—The training of rams for the artificial vagina with some observations on ram behaviour. *In* "Artificial Breeding of Sheep in Australia". (Ed. E. M. Roberts.) pp. 173–82. (Univ. of N.S.W.: Sydney.)

SARAPA, G. S. (1967).—The effect of technique of insemination on fertility in ewes. *Ovcevodstvo* **13**(8), 7–8.

SINCLAIR, A. N. (1957).—The effect of variation of mating, mating frequency and semen dose rate on conception in Merino sheep. *Aust. vet. J.* **33**, 88–91.

SNEDECOR, G. W. (1956).—"Statistical Methods." 5th Ed. p. 366. (Iowa St. Univ. Press: Ames.)

TERRILL, C. E. (1937).—Measurement of reproductive capacity as an aid in selection of rams of high fertility. *Rec. Proc. Am. Soc. Anim. Prod.* **30**, 311–16.

TERRILL, C. E. (1940).—Comparison of ram semen collection obtained by three different methods for artificial insemination. *Rec. Proc. Am. Soc. Anim. Prod.* **33**, 201–7.

WIGGINS, E. L., TERRILL, C. E., and EMIK, L. O. (1953).—Relationships between libido semen characteristics and fertility in range rams. *J. Anim. Sci.* **12**, 684–96.

Artificial Insemination in Domesticated
Birds

TRANSMISSION OF TYPE II (MAREK'S) LEUKOSIS WITH SEMEN FROM INFECTED ROOSTERS

Martin Sevoian

Type II (Marek's) leukosis has been reported to be caused by a filterable virus (Sevoian et al., 1962) and more recently a herpes-like virus (Churchill and Biggs, 1967; Nazerian et al., 1968). Transmission of this infection among chickens has been demonstrated with oral washings and feces (Witter and Burmester, 1967) and by the air borne route (Sevoian et al., 1963) from infected chickens. A more recent report

TABLE 1.—*Bioassay of semen and blood from infected roosters*

	Sample										Total	Controls
	1	2	3	4	5	6	7	8	9	10		
Trial 1												
Blood	−	+	+	+	+	+	+	−	+	+	8/10*	−
Semen	−	+	−	−	+	+	−	−	+	−	4/10	−
Trial 2												
Semen	−	+	+	+	+	−	+	+	−	+	7/10	−

* No. positive/total.

gave data indicating egg transmission (Sevoian, 1968) in support of earlier observation by Gibbs (1936) who found leukotic cells in the ovule of the ovary, in the tubes of the testes, and in the seminal and follicular fluids of infected roosters and hens respectively.

Trials reported herein indicate the infective status of semen from roosters infected with Type II leukosis.

MATERIALS AND METHODS

Donors of artificially collected semen were eight-month-old cross-bred roosters kept at the University farm under natural conditions. Approximately 0.5 cc. of semen was milked from each rooster into sterile centrifuge tubes. Each sample was diluted with 2 cc. of physiological saline containing 100 units of penicillin and 5 milligrams of streptomycin per cc. A bioassay was conducted in day-old S-line (susceptible) chicks wherein each of 5 chicks per semen sample received 0.5 cc. intraperitoneally. The chicks were placed in modified Horsfall-Bauer units for a period of 3 weeks when they were sacrificed and necropsied for lesions as previously described (Sevoian et al., 1962).

Blood from donor birds was drawn by venous puncture and bioassayed in S-line chicks (0.5 cc. of citrated blood per chick) as described above. Ten uninoculated control chicks were maintained in each trial.

RESULTS AND DISCUSSION

In Trial #1, four of ten semen samples were infective for S-line chicks (which developed tumors in the gonads and/or ganglia) whereas eight of ten blood samples from the same birds were infective. Every bird which had infective semen also had infective blood though four birds which had infective blood did not have positive semen (Table 1).

In Trial #2, seven of ten semen samples were infective for S-line chicks within a three-week incubation period. Typical tumorous lesions developed in the dorsal root ganglia or gonads or both.

It is not known whether the sperms themselves from the testes were infected or the vesicle fluid or both. It may be that the infection is not coming from either of these anatomical sites but rather from the cloaca through which the semen passes before being ejected through the vent where infection is known to exist and contamination could take place. In spite of the semen being infective, it is not known, further, whether such infection is carried mechanically to the ovum by the sperm. If sperms themselves are infected, the virus could then be incorporated within the zygote. The latter is presently being investigated by electron microscopy.

ACKNOWLEDGMENT

Grateful acknowledgment is given to Dr.

J. R. Smyth for collection of semen.

REFERENCES

Churchill, A. E., and P. M. Biggs, 1967. Agent of Marek's disease in tissue culture. Nature, 215: 528–530.

Gibbs, C. S., 1936. Observations and experiments with neurolymphomatosis and the leukotic diseases. Massachusetts Agricul. Exp. Sta. Bull. No. 337.

Nazerian, K., J. J. Solomon, R. L. Witter and B. R. Burmester, 1968. Studies on the etiology of Marek's disease. II. Finding of a herpesvirus in cell culture. Proc. Soc. Exp. Biol. Med. 127: 177–182.

Sevoian, M., 1968. Egg transmission studies of Type II leukosis infection (Marek's disease). Poultry Sci. 47: 1644–1646.

Sevoian, M., D. M. Chamberlain and F. T. Counter, 1962. Avian lymphomatosis. I. Experimental reproduction of the neural and visceral forms. Vet. Med. 57: 500–501.

Sevoian, M., D. M. Chamberlain and R. N. Larose, 1963. Avian lymphomatosis. V. Air-borne transmission. Avian Dis. 7: 102–105.

Witter, R. L., and B. R. Burmester, 1967. Transmission of Marek's disease with oral washings and feces from infected chickens. Proc. Soc. Exp. Biol. Med. 124: 59–62.

Frequency of Parthenogenesis in Chickens After Insemination With Irradiated Sperm

PATRICIA SARVELLA

INTRODUCTION

Parthenogenesis occurs in chickens at a low frequency and can give rise to either embryos or unorganized membranes (1). Various physical agents such as pricking (2) and hypotonic solutions (3) increased division in other types of eggs. Gynogenesis (fertilization by genetically inactivated sperm) occurred after treatment of spermatozoa by x-rays (see review by Beatty (4)). It was thought that irradiated viable sperm (motile although incapable of inseminating the egg) might cause the development of more parthenogenetic embryos in a parthenogenetic line of chicken.

MATERIALS AND METHODS

All treatments were given with a Gammacell 200 at the NASA's Goddard Space Flight Center at Greenbelt, Maryland. Semen was collected from the males, transported to the γ-source (about 15 minutes), and returned immediately after treatment to Beltsville and the females inseminated. These steps took less than 2 hours. Normal semen was also transported to determine the effect on viability.

The chickens used were a parthenogenetic line (mostly Dark Cornish type and will be referred to as Dark Cornish (1), and a White Leghorn line. The hens were virgin birds, hatched in July, sexed at 6 weeks, and placed in separate floor pens. At least 4 weeks prior to the experiments, the hens were moved to individual cages. Irradiations and inseminations were done weekly three different times.

Dosage levels in April and May, 1968 were given at a rate of 2×10^4 rads/min. (Table I). In 1969, the selected dose was 20 000 rads. One group of hens was inseminated with White Leghorn semen, and White Leghorn hens with Dark Cornish semen.

Eggs were incubated for 7–10 days when they were candled for live embryos. If there were none, the eggs were broken and examined macroscopically for parthenogenetic membranes and dead embryos. Parthenogenetic membranes were scored according to size: Class 0 had no visible membrane; Class 1, covered 10 % of the yolk; Class 2, about 25 % of the yolk; Class 3, 50 %, Class 4, 75 %; and Class 5, 100 %. Any visible blood in the membranes was also noted. The Dark Cornish eggs had intermediate frequencies of parthenogenetic membranes (10–40 %). White Leghorn eggs had a very low frequency of membranes (<1 %). The ratio of the number of membranes immediately before insemination was compared with the number of membranes from the same hens immediately after by means of chi-square tests. The types of membranes were compared in the same manner. Any living embryos were permitted to hatch, and the down color examined to detect any hybrids. White color is dominant, but in heterozygotes (hybrids) dark spots are visible from the Dark Cornish parent.

RESULTS

Preliminary Tests (1968)

To determine dose levels necessary to prevent fertility but allow insemination with motile sperm, White Leghorn sperm were irradiated at different doses (6000–

TABLE I

TESTING DOSAGE LEVELS TO PREVENT FERTILIZATION OF PARTHENOGENETIC DARK CORNISH CHICKENS. NUMBER OF EGGS WITH MEMBRANES BEFORE AND AFTER INSEMINATION, 1968

Dosage level (rads)	Ratio of membranes to total eggs		Chi-square test comparing	
	Before insemination	After insemination	Ratios	Distribution of membrane types
6000	55/166	18/39	ns	*a
8000	32/130	9/31	ns	*a
10 000	55/166	29/81	ns	*a
12 000	45/129	10/35	ns	ns
20 000	37/160	31/89	*a	+b
40 000	45/129	24/75	ns	+b
200 000	30/117	16/44	ns	+b
300 000	27/119	15/51	ns	ns

[a] * Represents $P < 0.05$.
[b] + Represents $P < 0.10$.

300 000 rads). The sperm given 6000–18 000 rads were examined under the micro-scope and were still very active—even 3 hours after semen collection. When given 10 000, 20 000, and 40 000 rads, the sperm were alive and very active after 15 minutes; at the end of 1.5 hours, some sperm were still active. The sperm at the 200 000 rad level moved slowly and were dead at the end of 1.5 hours, while the 300 000-rad dose immobilized almost all the sperm. Motility at the end of 15 minutes did not appear to be adversely affected by doses under 40 000 rads.

Eggs from the intermediate Dark Cornish hens were examined at the end of 7 days for parthenogenetic embryos and membranes (Table I). No embryos were observed. Only the 20 000-rad dose showed a significant increase of membranes. Surprisingly, the membranes were significantly more advanced (larger) in the lower three doses. Blood was observed in one egg each from the 6000, 10 000, and 20 000-rad treatments, but none in any eggs prior to insemination. The dose selected for the main experiment in 1969 was 20 000 rads.

White Leghorn Irradiated Semen (1969)

The frequencies and categories of membranes are given in Table II from the experiment in May and the replicate experiment in October, both before and after insemination. There were no differences between 3 different weeks of insemina-tion, therefore the data were combined. The number of membranes in the eggs after insemination compared with those of the same hens prior to insemination showed no difference in the eggs laid in May. The eggs from the replicate experi-ment in October had significantly more membranes than those immediately prior to insemination. More Class 1 membranes were observed in October than in May ($P < 0.01$).

The distribution of membrane types in the May eggs showed more eggs with Class 5 membranes and fewer with Class 1 membranes after insemination. Blood was observed in five membranes from the May eggs after insemination, but none prior. In October prior to insemination, six membranes had blood, but afterwards only three were observed; however, one embryo developed for about 3 days.

White Leghorn Transported Semen (1969)

Dark Cornish hens from the same flock were inseminated with nonirradiated, transported White Leghorn semen. The semen was still viable, and hybrid chicks hatched as detected by their down color (Table II). Therefore, viability was not affected by transporting the semen.

Dark Cornish Irradiated Semen (1969)

White Leghorn hens were inseminated with irradiated semen from Dark Cornish males. Only one egg had parthenogenetic development (Table II). This frequency was not significantly different from the percent ($<1\%$) prior to insemination.

TABLE II

NUMBER OF EGGS SHOWING PARTHENOGENESIS IN HENS INSEMINATED
WITH IRRADIATED SEMEN (20 000 RADS), 1969

	No. of hens	No. of eggs	No. of eggs with membrane types							Chi-square test comparing	
			0	1	2	3	4	5	Embryo	Ratios of eggs with membranes vs. those without	Distribution of membrane types
Dark Cornish hens inseminated irradiated White Leghorn semen											
May											
Before insemination	41	963	651	150	43	32	26	61	0	ns	**a
After insemination		419	279	34	21	15	15	55	0		
October											
Before insemination	39	213	111	45	8	9	11	29	0	*b	ns
After insemination		233	94	64	14	14	11	35	1		
Dark Cornish hens inseminated transported White Leghorn semen											
May											
Before insemination	4	182	136	17	7	6	2	14	0	**a	**a
After insemination		36	13	3	1	4	1	6	8		
October											
Before insemination	5	14	4	5	0	0	1	4	0	ns	+c
After insemination		28	6	3	0	0	1	9	9		
White Leghorn hens inseminated with irradiated Dark Cornish semen (May)											
After insemination	10	145	144	1							

a ** Represents $P < 0.01$.
b * Represents $P < 0.05$.
c + $P < 0.10$.

DISCUSSION

Membrane development differed in the parthenogenetic line of Dark Cornish chicken after insemination with irradiated semen compared with that prior to insemination. In the May experiment and low doses of 1968 the membranes were larger; whereas, in October and in 20 000 rads of 1968, the number of membranes was significantly increased. Variations in membrane frequencies may be due to environmental effects on the intermediate class of Dark Cornish eggs.[1] Since membrane classifications were based on macroscopic appearance, the larger number of membranes may reflect continued development of membranes already started on the microscopic level. Therefore, the two experiments may be the same.

Increased membrane development might be due to insemination and subsequent death of the embryo. If this occurred, then the White Leghorn hens inseminated with irradiated Dark Cornish semen should have had an increased frequency of membranes. Since this did not occur, the embryos and membranes observed in the Dark Cornish hens inseminated with the irradiated semen are most likely due to parthenogenetic development stimulated by the addition of this semen.

The irradiated sperm remained viable long enough to reach the infundibulum, since only 15 minutes to an hour is required (5). Transporting the sperm did not affect its capacity to fertilize the hens. Whether it remained alive long enough, or was capable of penetrating the egg is unknown. If it did, then it might be capable of acting as a triggering mechanism which could activate the eggs. If the sperm would have interacted with the egg, it might have stimulated parthenogenesis (gynogenesis) through the resulting physical and chemical changes in the egg surface (6). Spirin (7) speculated that stored m-RNA is unmasked and initiates protein synthesis. If these processes were activated by the irradiated sperm, then more parthenogenetic embryos would have been expected. Only one embryo was observed, therefore, embryo development was not affected. The irradiated sperm seemed to be most effective in causing more development of membranes (larger membranes and more membranes with blood). The processes, activation, stimulation, and organization, therefore, may be separate in the induction of parthenogenesis in chickens.

ACKNOWLEDGMENTS

I thank Mr. Frederick Gordon, Jr., Head Radiation Effects Section, Radiation Facility at NASA's Goddard Space Flight Center at Greenbelt, Maryland for doing the radiations. The stimulating conversations with Dr. M. W. Olsen were greatly appreciated. The help of Mr. Dean Montgomery and Mr. Leroy Brown is greatly appreciated.

REFERENCES

1. M. W. OLSEN, Frequency of parthenogenesis in chicken eggs. *J. Hered.* 57, 23–25 (1966).
2. E. BATAILLION, L'embryogenèse complète provoquée chez les Amphibiens par piqûre de l'oeuf vierge, larves parthènogènèseques de *Rana fusca. C. R. H. Acad. Sci.* 150, 996–998 (1910).
3. G. PINCUS and H. SHAPIRO, The comparative behavior of mammalian eggs *in vivo* and *in vitro*. VII. Further studies on the activation of rabbit eggs. *Proc. Amer. Phil. Soc.* 83, 631–647 (1940).

[1] P.A.Sarvella, Environmental effects on a parthenogenetic line of chickens. Unpublished results.

4. R. A. BEATTY, Gynogenesis in vertebrates: Fertilization by genetically inactivated spermatozoa. In *Effects of Ionizing Radiation on the Reproductive System.* (W. D. Carlson and F. X. Gassner, eds.), pp. 229–241. Pergamon Press, New York (1964).
5. T. E. ALLEN and G. W. GRIGG, Sperm transport in the fowl. *Aust. J. Agr. Res.* 8, 788–799 (1957).
6. A. MONROY, *Chemistry and Physiology of Fertilization.* Holt, Rinehart, and Winston, New York (1965).
7. S. SPIRIN, On "masked" forms of messenger RNA in early embryogenesis and in other differentiating systems. *Current Topics in Developmental Biology* 1, 1–38 (1966).

Observations on the Dilution
and Storage of Turkey Semen

J. B. K. CLARK, Ph.D., B.Sc., N.D.A., M.S.

Introduction

As a pre-requisite for high fertility in turkey hens, particularly of the broad-breasted strains, the employment of artificial techniques of insemination is indispensable. This paper describes the use of, and the results obtained from, the extensive use of undiluted and diluted semen which had been subjected to various periods of storage over an entire breeding period (13 weeks) in a commercial flock of turkeys. The problems of investigations of this nature, principally of cost and the rather limited amount of data that can be collected from the turkey hen in a given period of time, have been reviewed by Lorenz (1964) and the only published data on such experimentation are those of Millar and Garwood (1964) and Millar, Garwood and Hebert (1965), although these investigations did not include observations on semen storage. As far as can be ascertained, no data on the extensive use of diluted and stored turkey semen have been published hitherto, although Harper (1955), reporting on the use of undiluted and stored semen inseminated over a 16 week period, concluded that undiluted semen should be inseminated within one hour of collection.

There have been several reports dealing with the dilution and storage of turkey semen, based mainly on the results of single inseminations. Van Tienhoven, Steel and Duchaine (1958) reported some success with milk as a turkey semen diluent, although the fertility obtained with diluted semen was lower than that of undiluted semen. A Tyrode solution with added antibiotics or glycine gave the best fertility, although this was still about 15 per cent. below that obtained with undiluted semen. Wilcox and Shaffner (1960) reported that fertility of turkey semen was reduced substantially when diluted and stored in a sodium phosphate buffer containing fructose, antibiotics and turkey egg white. None of the reports cited indicated that there was a marked effect upon the hatchability of fertile eggs.

Materials and Methods

Experimental Design

The use of undiluted and immediately inseminated semen, diluted and immediately inseminated semen, and semen diluted and stored for six and 24 hour was investigated with two strains of broad-breasted turkey, a White (W) and Bronze (B) strain.

For each pen of hens within a strain, pooled semen from a group of 18 stags was used for each treatment. About 10 minutes elapsed during the collection of semen from a group and a further 20 minutes was taken to inseminate a pen of approximately 80 birds allocated to each treatment.

Eight pens of hens, (four of each strain), each containing approximately 80 hens initially, were allocated at random to the various treatments. A stag group rota system was devised so that the semen used on one pen of hens was used on a different pen of the same strain at the following insemination session. This largely eliminated any inter-stag group differences. Similarly, the times of insemination of the hens in any one pen at one session were rotated in order to minimise any differences in fertility that might have been attributable to the timing of insemination in relation to oviposition. Inseminations commenced at 3.30 p.m.

Housing

The pens in which the birds were kept were located in a pole barn and the hen and stag pens were situated on either side of a central corridor running the entire length of the barn. Twenty nests of the semi-trap variety were provided within each open pen of hens. No significance was attached to the use of this type of nest within the context of the experiment.

Birds

The age of all birds at the start of the experiment was between 32 and 35 weeks. All birds had been de-beaked at three weeks of age, had been vaccinated against Fowl Pest and were treated with "Tylan" (Injectable Elanco) against infectious sinusitis at point of lay. There were no apparent differences in extent of infection between the various pens, but during the course of the experiment any bird showing severe clinical symptoms was culled.

All hens were subjected to 8 hr. per day artificial light for 6 weeks before the experiment commenced. Oviposition was induced when the light was increased to 14 hours. The stags were subjected to a similar pattern for 9 wk. This was increased to 14 hours in order to induce semen production

Semen Collection, Dilution and Storage

Pooled samples of semen were collected by the usual method of digital massage around the cloacal region and the samples were aspirated into 10 ml. centrifuge tubes held in vacuum flasks at 16° C.; the apparatus being similar to that described by Cooper (1955). When diluted semen was required for storage, the tubes containing the diluted samples were placed in a 150 ml. beaker of water at 16° C. which was then placed in a refrigerator where it cooled slowly (circa. 7.5° C. per hr.) to 4° C. After the requisite storage time the tubes were allowed to warm slowly in the operator's hand during the insemination sessions.

In this experiment the volume of diluent added to the semen was arbitrarily decided at 1.5 vol. to 1 vol. of semen. The undiluted semen dosage rate employed was 0.03 ml. per hen and 0.075 ml. of the diluted semen was employed on the diluted treatments. Approximately equal numbers of spermatozoa were inseminated both within and between hen group treatments.

The composition of the diluent employed (*p*H 6.90, $\Delta - 0.63°$ C.) is shown in Table I. Its formulation was based on the findings of the work describing the biochemical composition òf fowl seminal plasma (Lake, 1966). In support of these findings Bajpai and Brown (1963), in a study on the effects of some diluents on turkey semen characteristics, demonstrated that sodium glutamate played a vital role in maintaining the motility of turkey spermatozoa. Polyhydric alcohols were added as their presence has been reported in the seminal plasma of both the bull (Clark, Graham, Lewis & Smith, 1967) and the domestic cock (Ahluwalia & Graham, 1963) and their beneficial effects on the preservations of viability and fertility of bovine semen have already been demonstrated (Clark, 1962 and Rajamannan, Graham & Smith, 1964). Gelatin was added in order to minimise sedimentation of spermatozoa during the insemination sessions.

TABLE I

COMPOSITION OF DILUENT (G. PER 100 ML. DISTILLED WATER)

L-glutamic acid, sodium salt. H$_2$O ...	2·5
Potassium citrate (K$_2$C$_r$H$_5$O$_7$. H$_2$O)...	0·25
Magnesium chloride (MgCl$_2$. H6$_2$O)	0·07
Glucose	0·3
m-inositol	0·1
D-mannitol	0·2
Sorbitol	0·2
Adonitol	0·1
Erythritol	0·05
Bacto-gelatin*	0·25
Oxytetracycline	0·009
Dihydrostreptomycin sulphate ...	0·009

*Difco Labs. Inc., Detroit, Mich., U.S.A.

Inseminations

Inseminations were carried out with a Wasser-Nechmad A.I syringe* to which a glass pipette was fitted with a short piece of rubber tubing. One pipette was used for each pen of hens. Three initial inseminations were made at intervals of seven days and thereafter the interval was increased to 14 days until the completion of the experiment.

Broody hens, always a problem in turkey breeding experiments, were removed immediately on detection and placed in broody coops (one within each pen of hens) and re-inseminated within one week; those due for insemination the following week were again inseminated while the others awaited their allotted time.

Eggs

Eggs were collected from the second day after the first insemination and daily thereafter. They were sterilised and incubated in accordance with routine commercial practice. All abnormal eggs were discarded. Incubated eggs were candled after 24 days to detect fertile eggs and dead embryos.

The fertility and hatch data were analysed by routine statistical methods. Tests of significance were carried out on pen totals only and no attempt was made to determine within-pen variance. Compari-

---

* Alfred Cox Ltd., Coulsdon, Surrey.

TABLE II

SUMMARY OF RESULTS

Breed		Broad-breasted white		
Group	W1	W2	W3	W4
Dose (ml.)	0·03	0·075	0·075	0·075
Dilution	Undiluted	1 + 1·5	1 + 1·5	1 + 1·5
Storage (hour)	0	0	6	24
Insemination pattern	A.I. three times at 7 day intervals and then every 14th day to total of 13 weeks			
No. hens at start of experiment	81	83	80	79
Mortality during experiment	28	18	21	19
Eggs laid—total	2,817	3,136	2,902	2,897
eggs per week per ♀	3·05	3·11	3·10	3·04
Eggs set—total	2,671	3,024	2,740	2,725
eggs per week per ♀	2·85	2·97	2·91	2·82
Per cent fertile (of eggs set)	69·4	76·2	46·7	30·0
Dead germs (of eggs set)	2·6	2·1	1·6	1·5
Dead-in-shell (of eggs set)	7·9	7·2	5·4	2·7
Dead poults (of eggs in hatcher)	0·44	0·75	2·3	0·87
Poults helped out (of eggs in hatcher)	5·5	4·5	4·6	7·2
Per cent. hatch of fertile eggs	88·6	90·6	87·5	91·0
Per cent. hatch of all eggs set	61·3	69·1	40·9	27·1
Per cent first quality poults (of poults hatched)	89·3	91·5	90·3	87·1
Per cent. reject poults (of poults hatched)	4·0	2·8	2·8	4·0
First quality poults/hen/total	20·6	24·5	14·2	8·8
First quality poults/hen/week	1·71	2·04	1·18	0·73
First quality poults—per cent. difference from controls associated with treatment	Control	+19·1	−31·3	−57·7

Breed		Broad-breasted bronze			
Group		B1	B2	B3	B4
Dose (ml.)		0·03	0·075	0·075	0·075
Dilution		Undiluted	1+1·5	1 + 1·5	1 + 1·5
Storage (hour)		0	0	6	24
Insemination pattern		A.I. three times at 7 day intervals and then every 14th day to total of 13 weeks			
No. of hens at start of experiment		80	80	80	78
Mortality during experiment		7	8	12	16
Eggs laid—total		3,199	3,159	3,039	2,987
eggs per week per ♀		3·23	3·17	3·11	3·19
Eggs set—total		3,042	2,943	2,885	2,855
eggs per week per♀		3·04	2·94	2·93	3·03
Per cent. fertile (of eggs set)		71·9	78·5	47·8	35·2
Dead germs (of eggs set)		2·7	3·5	2·1	1·0
Dead-in-shell (of eggs set)		8·8	8·5	5·6	3·3
Dead poults (of eggs in hatcher)		0·42	0·26	0·37	0·50
Poults helped out (of eggs in hatcher)		7·1	7·2	7·2	7·6
Per cent. hatch of fertile eggs		87·8	89·6	88·2	90·7
Per cent. hatch of all eggs set		63·7	72·8	41·9	32·0
Per cent first quality poults (of poults hatched)		88·6	85·5	88·6	88·4
Per cent. reject poults (of poults hatched)		2·8	2·6	2·8	2·7
First quality poults/hen/total		22·1	23·9	14·2	11·2
First quality poults/hen/week		1·84	1·99	1·18	0·93
First quality poults—per cent. difference from controls associated with treatment		Control	+8·1	−35·8	−49·4

Breed

<table>
<tr><td></td><td colspan="4" align="center">Combined (W + B)</td></tr>
<tr><td>Group</td><td>1</td><td>2</td><td>3</td><td>4</td></tr>
<tr><td>Dose (ml.) … … … …</td><td>0·03</td><td>0·075</td><td>0·075</td><td>0·075</td></tr>
<tr><td>Dilution … … … …</td><td>Undiluted</td><td>1 + 1·5</td><td>1 + 1·5</td><td>1 + 1·5</td></tr>
<tr><td>Storage (hour) … … …</td><td>0</td><td>0</td><td>6</td><td>24</td></tr>
<tr><td>Insemination pattern … …</td><td colspan="4">A.I. three times at 7 day intervals and then every 14th day to total of 13 weeks</td></tr>
<tr><td>No. of hens at start of experiment …</td><td>161</td><td>163</td><td>160</td><td>157</td></tr>
<tr><td>Mortality during experiment …</td><td>35</td><td>26</td><td>33</td><td>35</td></tr>
<tr><td>Eggs laid—total … …</td><td>6,016</td><td>6,295</td><td>5,941</td><td>5,884</td></tr>
<tr><td>eggs per week per ♀ …</td><td>3·14</td><td>3·14</td><td>3·10</td><td>3·10</td></tr>
<tr><td>Eggs set—total … …</td><td>5,713</td><td>5,967</td><td>5,625</td><td>5,580</td></tr>
<tr><td>eggs per week ♀ …</td><td>2·95</td><td>2·95</td><td>2·92</td><td>2·92</td></tr>
<tr><td>Per cent. fertile (of eggs set) …</td><td>70·8</td><td>77·3</td><td>47·3</td><td>32·6</td></tr>
<tr><td>Dead germs (of eggs set) …</td><td>2·7</td><td>2·8</td><td>1·8</td><td>1·3</td></tr>
<tr><td>Dead-in-shell (of eggs set) …</td><td>8·4</td><td>7·8</td><td>5·5</td><td>3·0</td></tr>
<tr><td>Dead poults (of eggs in hatcher) …</td><td>0·43</td><td>0·50</td><td>1·29</td><td>0·67</td></tr>
<tr><td>Poults helped out (of eggs in hatcher)</td><td>6·4</td><td>5·8</td><td>6·0</td><td>7·4</td></tr>
<tr><td>Per cent. hatch of fertile eggs … …</td><td>88·2</td><td>90·1</td><td>87·9</td><td>90·8</td></tr>
<tr><td>Per cent. hatch of all eggs set …</td><td>62·6</td><td>70·9</td><td>41·4</td><td>29·6</td></tr>
<tr><td>Per cent. first quality poults (of poults hatched)</td><td>89·0</td><td>88·4</td><td>89·5</td><td>87·8</td></tr>
<tr><td>Per cent. reject poults (of poults hatched) …</td><td>3·4</td><td>2·7</td><td>2·8</td><td>3·2</td></tr>
<tr><td>First quality poults/hen/total … …</td><td>21·4</td><td>24·2</td><td>14·2</td><td>10·0</td></tr>
<tr><td>First quality poults/hen/week. … …</td><td>1·78</td><td>2·02</td><td>1·18</td><td>0·83</td></tr>
<tr><td>First quality poults—per cent. difference from controls associated with treatment … … …</td><td>Control</td><td>+13·2</td><td>−33·7</td><td>−53·5</td></tr>
</table>

sons of egg laying performance, fertility of eggs set, and poult production by the various treatments, were made by variance analysis. All other statistical comparisons were made by computations of chi square.

Results

A summary of all the recorded data is presented in Table II. In this table it should be noted that the fertility data presented cover the duration of the experiment, namely thirteen weeks. However, due to an oversight, fertile eggs produced during the first week were transferred, after the 24 day candling, to the hatching compartments of the incubators without regard to their pens of origin. Thus, the results cited for hatch exclude those for the first week. The numbers of eggs "lost" in this manner were 28, 27, 2 and 16 from Groups W1, 2, 3 and 4 respectively and 32, 10, 19 and 6 from Groups B1, 2, 3 and 4 respectively.

Hen Mortality

During the course of the experiment there was a high incidence of mortality (including hens culled). This incidence was almost twice as high among the White hens (26.6 per cent.) as compared to the Bronze hens (13.5 per cent.). This difference attained high statistical significance ($p < 0.001$). There were no statistically significant differences in mortality rates that could be associated with treatments.

Egg Production

The difference in the number of eggs laid over the experimental period by the hens receiving undiluted and diluted semen was not statistically significant ($p > 0.1$). However, overall, the Bronze hens laid more eggs per hen than the White hens ($p = 0.10$). There were indications that maximum egg production of the hens that received the diluted semen occurred a little later than in those hens that received the undiluted semen, although whether this was cause and effect could not be ascertained.

Fertility

From Table II it will be observed that the Bronze hens as well as laying more eggs, laid a statistically higher proportion of fertile eggs ($p < 0.05$) than the White hens.

Fig. 1 illustrates a marked decline in fertility associated with storage of semen. However, for the first few weeks of the experiment, the pattern of fertility was similar for all the diluted semen treatments, *i.e.* there was a gradual build-up in fertility up to the third week which contrasted quite markedly with the undiluted semen treatments in which an initial

210

high fertility was followed by a gradual decline. A comparison of the respective egg fertility figures between the diluted and the undiluted semen groups over weeks 1 to 4, 5 to 8 and 9 to 13 showed that the undiluted groups (W1 + B1) commenced at 84.6 per cent. in the first period, fell to 78.1 per cent. during the second and terminated at 51.0 per cent. The corresponding figures for the diluted groups (W2 + B2) were 81.9 per cent., 82.7 per cent. and 69.0 per cent. respectively. The difference in fertility between the undiluted groups (84.6 per cent.) and that of the diluted groups (81.9 per cent.) over the first four-weekly period was statistically significant ($p < 0.05$). There was no evidence of any statistically significant interaction between strain of bird and treatment. During the entire period of the experiment, the combined fertility obtained with diluted and immediately inseminated semen was significantly greater (77.3 per cent. vs. 70.8 per cent.; $p < 0.001$) than that obtained with undiluted semen (Table II).

Hatchability
With regard to fecundity, a significantly higher number of poults ($p < 0.01$) was hatched from eggs produced by hens associated with diluent and inseminated immediately, than was hatched from hens inseminated with undiluted semen. A statistically significantly greater number of White poults was rejected than Bronze immediately after hatching ($p < 0.05$) and, between treatments, a significantly greater number of poults from the undiluted groups was culled than from the undiluted groups ($p < 0.10$).

Discussion
It has been demonstrated that diluted turkey semen can result in a very satisfactory level of poult production when used on a large scale over an entire breeding season. However, it is apparent that semen should be used as soon as possible after collection and dilution.

The number of hens which died in all groups during the course of this investigation was unusually high and was attributed by the owner to the dry summer. The number of eggs laid was probably a reflection of this explanation and also of a high incidence of broodiness. In particular, it was noted that the White hens were more likely to die than the Bronze hens and were therefore probably of less sound physical constitution.

Clearly, the cumulative fertility level after six- and 24-hour storage is uneconomic. However, it was encouraging to note that even after such prolonged

211

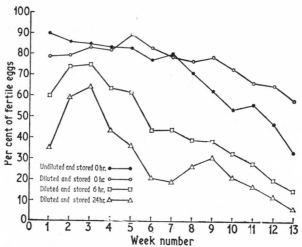

FIG. 1.—The effect of dilution and storage of semen on fertility (W and B groups combined).

semen storage, fertility at week 3 (Fig. 1) was quite significant (75 per cent. and 67 per cent. respectively) and these results may aid further research. In the present study, the results obtained from the use of diluted and undiluted semen, inseminated immediately, and measured by the various parameters recorded in Table II raise several interesting points.

Since the insemination doses, in terms of numbers of spermatozoa, were approximately equal for all treatments the fertility "build-up" phenomenon is difficult to explain. There may have been an initial adverse diluent-genital tract interaction which was eventually overcome, but this point could be an important factor in the design of experiments to evaluate semen diluents, e.g. a single challenge with diluted semen may not necessarily reveal the true potential of the diluent. In a recent study on the use of carbon dioxide diluents for turkey semen, Bajpai and Brown (1967) concluded also that fertility trials should be conducted over an entire breeding season, or, if single inseminations are to be employed, they should be done also during the latter half of the season.

It is interesting to note, too, (Table II) that if the proportion of eggs pipping and hatching is an indication of poult virility, then it may possibly be concluded that poults from eggs out of hens inseminated with diluted semen are stronger than those from eggs out of hens inseminated with undiluted semen. This difference, associated with diluent, was statistically significant (p<0.05).

In conclusion, it should be stressed that the results of this experiment, albeit carried out on a large number of birds, relate to one experiment carried out at one centre only. Further experimental evidence on the use of diluted turkey semen (Clark, unpublished data) has indicated that the benefits to be derived from the use of diluent and immediate insemination tend to be rather variable and may possibly be inversely associated with the employment of good management techniques. However, if the data presented are studied in the light of the results obtained from the use of diminishing semen doses (Millar & Garwood, 1964; Millar *et al.*, 1965), then it does seem likely that considerable economic gain could be derived from the use of diluent, both in the direction of increased poult production and a concomitant decrease in the number of stags required.

Acknowledgments.—The author is indebted to Mr. W. H. G. Lloyd, Manager at Brewery House Farm, Middle Wallop, Hampshire, and to his staff for their interest and co-operation in carrying out this trial. He is indebted also to Miss S. V. Cunliffe, Head of the Statistics Department, Arthur Guinness, Son & Co. Ltd., Park Royal, London, N.W.10, for the statistical analyses of the data and their interpretation. Thanks also are due to Miss P. Hayden for her assistance in the preparation of the typescript.

References

AHLUWALIA. B. S., & GRAHAM, E. F. (1963). *Poult. Sci.* **42.** 1,251 (abstr.).

BAJPAI, P. K., & BROWN, K. I. (1963). *Ibid.* **42.** 882.

———, & ———. (1967) *Ibid.* 46. 599.

CLARK, J. B. K. (1962). Ph.D. Thesis, University of Minnesota.

———, GRAHAM. E. F., LEWIS, B. A., & SMITH, F. (1967). *J. Reprod. Fert.* **13.** 189.

HARPER, J. A. (1955). *Poult. Sci.* **34.** 1,289.

LAKE, P. E. (1966). In "Advances in Reproductive Physiology." Ed. A. McLaren. Vol. 1. P. 93. Logos Press, London.

LORENZ, F. W. (1964). *Proc. Vth Intl. Congr. Anim. Reprod. Artif. Insem., Trento.* **4.** 7.

MILLAR, P. G., & GARWOOD, F. E. (1964). *Vet. Rec.* **76.** 624.

———, ———, & HEBERT, C. NANCY (1965). *Ibid.* **77.** 130.

RAJAMANNAN, H. J., GRAHAM, E. F., & SMITH, F. (1964). *Proc. Vth Intl. Congr. Anim. Reprod. Artif. Insem., Trento.* **4.** 392.

VAN TIENHOVEN, A., STEEL, R. G. D., & DUCHAINE, S. A. (1958). *Poult. Sci.* **37.** 47.

WILCOX, F. H., & SHAFFNER, C. S. (1960). *Ibid.* **39.** 1,580.

Method and Frequency of Artificial Insemination and Turkey Fertility

KARL E. NESTOR AND KEITH I. BROWN

L OW fertility is still a serious problem in producing turkey hatching eggs even though most turkeys are artificially inseminated. Generally, the fertility of turkey eggs is relatively high at the beginning of the breeding season and then declines as the season progresses.

Several factors may be responsible for the seasonal decline in fertility. Among these are faulty insemination techniques, as shown by Ogasawara and Rooney (1966), and mechanical spread of infectious organisms from hen to hen by the insemination technique.

Many turkey breeders and turkey hatching egg producers are now using a disposable plastic tube for insemination in order to prevent spread of vaginal infection. Although the use of the tube method of insemination has become an established practice commercially, there has been little experimental evidence to show that it is a superior method. In a preliminary report of the present work, Nestor and Brown (1966) observed that the tube method of insemination gave higher fertility than the syringe method. Bajpai and Brown (1964) compared the syringe and rod methods of insemination. Fertility obtained with the two methods of insemination was identical.

Burrows and Marsden (1938) inseminated turkeys repeatedly at intervals of 1, 2, 3, and 4 weeks and found no apparent tendency for fertility to decline with increasing length of interval between successive inseminations. McCartney (1952) found that increasing the insemination interval from 2 to 4 weeks resulted in a highly significant decrease in fertility, but in a later study (1954) observed no significant difference in fertility between intervals of 2 and 3 weeks. More recent work (Bajpai and Brown, 1964; Nestor and Brown, 1966; and Ogasawara and Rooney,

214

1966) indicates that fertility is increased by weekly inseminations in comparison to bi-weekly inseminations, especially late in the laying season.

The purpose of this experiment was to determine the influence of method and frequency of insemination on turkey fertility.

MATERIALS AND METHODS

The methods of insemination compared in this experiment were the syringe, tube, and glass rod.

Semen was inseminated by means of a 0.25 cc. glass syringe (B.D. Yale with glass Luer tip) with the syringe method. The tube method of insemination used in this experiment consisted of attaching a rigid plastic tube (5 mm. $\times$ .4 cc. $\times$ 10.16 cm.) to a section of plastic tubing, dipping the tube into semen, and blowing the semen into the oviduct by mouth. A different tube was used for each hen. The tubes were washed and re-used. They were washed in water containing detergent and then allowed to soak in a 95% ethyl alcohol solution for at least one day. After soaking, they were dried and re-used.

The glass rod method was similar to the method described by Bajpai and Brown (1964). A common glass rod (approximately 3.0 mm. $\times$ 15 cm.) was used to inseminate all hens in a group in this study. A concave cup was formed on one end of the rod by heating. The end with the depression was dipped into the semen and then inserted in the oviduct and wiped clean.

The syringe and rod methods would be conducive to spread of infectious organisms from hen to hen since repeated inseminations were made without sterilization. The posssibility was minimized with the tube method.

The hens in all trials were from different flocks of a strain selected for and exhibiting high egg production. This strain was initiated in 1960 from a randombred control population (McCartney, 1964) and has changed very little in body weight since that time. Most of the comparisons were made during hot weather late in the laying season when the fertility level is normally low.

Pooled semen from 20 to 30 males was divided into aliquots. A different aliquot was used with each method of insemination. No effort was made to keep constant the amount of semen inseminated per hen with the different methods of insemination. However, an excessive amount of semen (in excess of 0.02 cc. per hen) was used with the tube and syringe methods of insemination. Semen was collected and held at 15°C. during insemination.

Eggs were set at weekly intervals. They were candled on the seventh day of incubation. Eggs classified as infertiles were broken open and examined macroscopically in order to check for the presence of early dead embryos which could not be determined by candling.

The statistical significance of treatment differences in fertility and hatchability was estimated by analysis of variance. Fertility and hatchability were considered as traits of the hen so the error term was based on the variance between hens within treatments. The use of pooled semen should randomize the effect of males. Percentage values were converted to arcsine $\sqrt{\text{percentage}}$ prior to analysis.

RESULTS AND DISCUSSION

The percent fertility obtained with various treatments is summarized in Table 1. Fertility obtained by the use of the tube method was consistently higher than that obtained with the other two methods. However, the differences among methods of insemination were significant (P < .05) only in comparisons made very late in the laying season (18 to 27 weeks and 28 to 36

215

Method of insem.	Freq. of insem.	Weeks of lay			
		10–15	16–21	18–27	28–36
		% Fertility			
Syringe	Weekly		74 (12/107)		40 (11/280)[2]
Tube	Weekly	76 (39/743)[1]	86 (17/199)	86 (18/625)[2,3]	69 (12/231)
Rod	Weekly	64 (37/734)	66 (16/187)	68 (17/572)	39 (10/265)
Tube	Bi-Weekly	78 (40/790)		64 (17/590)	
Rod	Bi-Weekly	65 (41/812)		56 (17/626)	

[1] Numbers in parenthesis refer to number of hens/numbers of eggs on which the fertility averages were based.
[2] Differences between methods were significant (P<.01).
[3] Differences between frequency of insemination were significant (P<.05).

weeks). The syringe and rod methods gave similar fertility. There was no significant difference in hatchability of fertile eggs between treatments in any trial.

The superiority of the tube method may have been due to several factors. Among these are: (1) prevention of spread of infectious organisms by this method; (2) oxygenation of the semen by the use of the tube method; and (3) fewer hens being completely infertile with the tube method because of presence of semen on the outside of the tube as well as being blown in the oviduct with more force resulting in a wider distribution of the semen in the oviduct.

In order to determine whether the first of the above possible explanations was a factor in higher fertility obtained with the tube method, one group of 64 hens was inseminated using a common tube for all hens and a similar group was inseminated with a clean tube for each hen. Weekly inseminations were made over a twelve-week period. There was no significant difference in fertility and hatchability (Table 2). This indicates that something other than prevention of spread of infectious organisms was responsible for the superiority of the tube method. This agrees with the results of Ogasawara and Rooney (1966) who found that treatments of hens with an-

tibiotics in a low fertility flock did not increase fertility. They postulated that the low fertility of this flock was the result of insufficient numbers of spermatozoa being inseminated rather than from a reaction to an unidentified pathogenic agent.

Aeration of semen at the time of insemination may have resulted in the increased fertility obtained with the tube method. However, Harper (1965) found that aeration of semen for 15, 60 and 120 minutes following collection did not affect the fertilizing capacity of spermatozoa. Schindler and Nevo (1962) found that, depending on dilution, cock spermatozoa became inactive after a period of from 2 to 30 minutes due to lack of ozygen. Thus it is possible that Harper's aerated samples became inactive, or largely so, after aeration was discontinued before insemination and therefore did not differ from non-aerated samples in motility. Since turkey semen is more concentrated than cock semen, the inactivation of turkey spermatozoa as the result of lack of

TABLE 2.—*The effect of using a common tube for all hens*

Treatment	No. eggs set	Percent fertility	% Hatchability of fertile eggs
Common Tube	2,057	87.3	63.2
Tubes Changed	1,992	88.4	67.6

TABLE 3.—*Fertility of eggs according to days following insemination*

	Days after insemination						
	2	3	4	5	6	7	8
No. Eggs	513	499	445	542	543	508	527
Percent Fertility	69	71	70	66	64	65	61

oxygen would proceed at a more rapid rate. Inactivated cock spermatozoa can be reactivated by addition of oxygen (Schindler and Nevo, 1962). The oxygenation occurring with insemination by the tube method could have increased the motility at the time when motility is probably most important in fertilization and thus increased fertility.

The spreading of semen over a larger area of the vagina due to the pressure involved in blowing the semen into the oviduct could also have been an important factor in the higher fertility obtained with the tube method. This, along with the semen adhering to the outside of the tube, probably reduced the chance of hens being completely infertile as the result of inadequate numbers of spermatozoa. The volume of semen on the outside of the tube was probably as great as the volume inseminated with the rod method.

Weekly inseminations resulted in higher fertility (P < .05) than bi-weekly inseminations in a fertility trial conducted during the 18th to 27th weeks of lay (Table 1). Such a difference was not evident during the 10th to 15th weeks of lay. This indicates that frequency of insemination is more important late in the laying season. The fertility obtained with weekly inseminations later in the laying period (18 to 27 weeks) was actually slightly higher than corresponding fertility obtained earlier (19 to 15 weeks). However, inseminations every two weeks were not capable of maintaining the same level of fertility.

The difference in results obtained with frequency of insemination between the ear-lier work and more recent experiments may be explained by a difference in body weight of the strains involved since large gains in body weight have been made by commercial turkey breeders in the last 10 to 12 years. Ogasawara *et al.* (1963) found a negative genetic correlation between body weight during the growing season and level of fertility as well as the ability to maintain fertility following insemination.

The question arose whether inseminating more frequently than once a week might increase fertility late in the laying season. To answer this, data were collected on the fertility obtained in eggs laid from 2 through 8 days following insemination. Due to time involved in egg formation, eggs are not normally fertilized until the second day following insemination. Thus, the second day following insemination would represent the first day in which eggs were fertilized by that insemination.

Data collected on 216 hens over a nine-week period (during the 18th to 26th weeks of production) are presented in Table 3. Fertility reached a peak three days after insemination and then declined. The fertility of eggs laid eight days after insemination was ten percent less than that obtained on the third day following insemination. These results suggest that insemination more frequently than once per week would improve fertility late in the season.

SUMMARY

The tube method of insemination resulted in consistently higher fertility than either the glass rod or syringe methods. The use of a common tube for all hens or a clean tube for each hen gave similar fertility, suggesting that prevention of spread of infectious organisms was not a factor in the superiority of the tube method. The syringe and rod methods of insemination gave similar fertility. Method of insemination had no influence on hatchability of fertile eggs.

More frequent inseminations resulted in higher fertility late in the laying season. There was no significant difference in fertility obtained between weekly and bi-weekly insemination when data were collected from the tenth to fifteenth weeks of lay. A significantly higher level of fertility was obtained with weekly inseminations from the 18th to 27th weeks of lay.

REFERENCES

Bajpai, P. K., and K. I. Brown, 1964. Observations on turkey fertility. Ohio Report, 49: 76–77.

Burrows, W. H., and S. J. Marsden, 1938. Artificial breeding of turkeys. Poultry Sci. 17: 408–411.

Harper, J. A., 1965. Fertility of turkey eggs as related to method of collecting and aeration of semen. Poultry Sci. 44: 726–731.

McCartney, M. G., 1952. The physiology of reproduction in turkeys. 3. Effect of frequency of mating and semen dosage on fertility and hatchability. Poultry Sci. 31: 878–881.

McCartney, M. G., 1954. The physiology of reproduction in turkeys. 4. Relation of frequency of mating and semen dosage to reproductive performance. Poultry Sci. 33: 390–391.

McCartney, M. G., 1964. A randombred control population of turkeys. Poultry Sci. 43: 739–744.

Nestor, K. E., and K. I. Brown, 1966. Method and frequency of artificial insemination influence turkey fertility. Ohio Report, 50: 74.

Ogasawara, F. X., and W. F. Rooney, 1966. Artificial insemination and fertility in turkeys. British Poultry Sci. 7: 77–82.

Ogasawara, F. X., H. Abplanalp and V. S. Asmundson, 1963. Effect of selection for body weight and reproduction in turkey hens. Poultry Sci. 42: 838–842.

Schindler, H., and A. Nevo, 1962. Reversible inactivation and agglutination of fowl and bull spermatozoa under anaerobic conditions. J. Reprod. Fertil. 4: 251–265.

Bacterial Flora of Semen and Contamination of the Reproductive Organs of the Hen following Artificial Insemination

M. PEREK, M. ELIAN AND E. D. HELLER

ARTIFICIAL INSEMINATION (A.I.) OF fowls is used widely on commercial farms in Israel. This method is adopted because it permits more efficient use of males of proven genetic stock and ensures a better fertilization rate, as reported by Cooper (1955) and by Lutzenberg and Doehl (1956). It also facilitates the evaluation of semen for the elimination of sterile males (Perek, 1966) and it is the only system available for obtaining hatching eggs from a cage-kept flock and for keeping exact records. However, most farmers report a sharp decrease in egg fertility after inseminations over a period of 3 to 6 months (sometimes 50% and less) in spite of the fact that the motility and concentration of spermatozoa in the semen was normal. No such decline in fertility was observed during the same period in similar flocks kept on deep litter. It is suggested by the authors that lowered fertility might be the result of repeated contamination of the oviducts of the hens by the cloacal flora in the semen of the milked cockerels.

The purpose of the present work was to identify the microflora prevailing in the semen obtained from cockerels and to study the possible effect on the reproductive tract of the hen.

MATERIALS AND METHODS

Semen of cockerels was collected by the method of Burrows and Quinn (1939) into individual sterile tubes. Semen collected, after first cleansing the exterior of the cloaca, from cockerels on our own farm was sown within 15 minutes on the various media. Samples taken from other farms were stored in ice for 1 to 2 hours before being sown. 0·05 ml. of each semen sample was sown on the following media:

Isolation media: MacConkey agar, SS agar, Chapman stone, tomato juice agar, enteroccoci confirmatory agar, Sabouraud dextrose agar with added penicillin, streptomycin and chloramphenicol, PPLO agar and blood agar.

Enrichment media: Selenite broth, azide dextrose broth, Brewer thioglycollate and MacConkey broth.

Bacterial Counts

Bacterial counts of semen were performed on the differential media by adequately diluting the semen in Ringer's saline solution ($NaH_4PO_4.2H_2O.Na_2$

HPO$_4$·7H$_2$O in 0·8% NaCl, pH 7·0). The organisms added to the semen were grown on adequate media in Roux flasks, washed in Ringer's saline solution, then centrifuged three times at 15 g. for 30 minutes. The sediment was taken in Ringer's saline solution and the bacterial cell concentration was determined by nephelometry.

Bacterial Examination of Organs

The hens were killed and the reproductive organs, liver, spleen and gall bladder were recovered and dissected aseptically. Each section of the oviduct was placed in a sterile petri plate from which swabs were taken and sown on appropriate media. A Beckman Zeromatic II was used to take pH readings of the various parts of the oviducts within 10 minutes of death.

Identification of Micro-organisms

Enterobacteriaceae were identified by the biochemical and serological methods recommended by Edwards and Ewing (1964). Groupings of streptococci were performed according to Deibel (1964), Simpson-Nowlan and Deibel (1967), Bergey's Manual (1957) and Topley and Wilson (1964). Classification of the other organisms were determined biochemically and serologically according to Bergey's Manual (1957) and Topley and Wilson (1964). Serological tests were made with antisera sets from Difco Laboratories, U.S.A. *E. coli* strains were phage-typed after isolation from semen and organs by the phage typing laboratory of the Department of Health, Jerusalem. *M. gallisepticum* was identified following culturing and tests recommended by Yoder (1965).

Experiment 1

The semen of 103 cockerels kept in the poultry house of the Department of Poultry Science and 361 cockerels on 7 commercial farms was examined and the bacterial flora identified. In addition, the organisms were counted in 250 specimens of semen collected from 125 cockerels; 20 cockerels, whose semen repeatedly contained the same organisms, were killed and the testes, liver, spleen and cloaca examined bacteriologically.

Experiment 2

A total of 78 hens were divided into 7 groups and inseminated with 0·05 ml. of semen at 2-day intervals as follows: 6 hens 4 times, 6 hens 6 times, 30 hens 10 times, 10 hens 20 times, 10 hens 30 times, and 10 hens 40 times. The seventh group of 6 hens (controls) received intrauterine instillations 40 times

with Ringer's saline solution. At the end of each period of insemination each group was killed 4–6 days after the last insemination and the reproductive organs dissected for bacteriological examinations.

Experiment 3

Eighty hens divided into 8 equal groups were inseminated with 0·05 ml. of semen with the following concentrations of organisms added. Three groups received *E. coli* at 1 × 10^6, 10 × 10^6 and 50 × 10^6 respectively. and three groups received similar concentrations of group D streptococci. Group 7 received semen alone and group 8 served as controls, receiving Ringer's saline solution only. All the groups were inseminated 15 times at 4-day intervals. All the hens were killed 4 to 6 days after the last insemination and their reproductive organs examined bacteriologically.

Experiment 4

A total of 42 hens were divided into 7 equal groups of which 6 were treated by intrauterine injections with suspensions of 6 bacterial species. Each of the suspensions contained 0·5 × 10^6 *E. coli*, group D streptococci, *Strep. alpha haemolyticus*, klebsiella, proteus sp., *C. albicans*, in 0·05 ml. of Ringer's saline, respectively. Group 7 received Ringer's saline only. Each group was treated 10 times at 4-day intervals. The hens were killed 4 days following the last treatment and their oviducts, liver and spleen examined bacteriologically.

RESULTS

Semen Flora

Table I demonstrates the distribution of various bacterial species in the semen of 464 cockerels. A total of 360 samples were examined once only, while 103 cockerels were examined 5 times over a period of 6 months. The same bacterial species was found repeatedly in each of the individual semen samples. As seen from Table I, *E. coli* and group D streptococci were prevalent together in most of the samples, each appearing 248 times, while *C. albicans*, proteus sp., *Strep. alpha haemolyticus*, klebsiella, *P. aeruginosa*, *Mycoplasma* group and members of Arizona group were isolated from 60, 59, 37, 29, 8, 3 and 1 sample, respectively. Colonies of lactobacilli, diphtheroids and *Staph. albus* (non-haemolytic) found in a few samples were disregarded and not included in the table.

and end of the test, which lasted 6 months. The same types were obtained persistently from the semen of each individual cockerel.

TABLE I

BACTERIAL FLORA IN SEMEN SAMPLES FROM 464 COCKERELS

Farm	A	B	C	D	E	F	G	Uni-versity Farm	Total
No. of Cockerels	49	42	50	47	50	46	77	103	464

Micro-organisms isolated									Totals	% of infections
Escherichia coli	20	25	27	27	8	14	42	85	248	35·9
Group D streptococci	15	29	37	31	30	30	30	46	248	35·9
Candida albicans	7	—	1	1	2	17	23	9	60	8·7
Proteus sp.	11	4	—	4	4	7	1	28	59	8·5
Streptococcus alpha haemolyticus	—	—	—	—	5	—	3	29	37	5·3
Klebsiella	7	2	—	—	6	5	—	4	24	3·5
Pseudomonas	—	—	—	—	—	—	2	6	8	1·2
Clostridia	—	—	—	—	—	3	—	—	3	0·4
Mycoplasma gallisepticum	—	—	—	—	—	—	—	3	3	0·4
Arizona group	—	—	—	—	1	—	—	—	1	0·1

A plate count of the total bacterial flora per ml. of semen was performed at random from 250 samples. Some samples contained only a few bacterial cells (10^1), others reached 10^6, while half of the samples were found in the range of 10^3 counts.

Since repeated tests of the semen proved that each of the cockerels shed its particular organisms throughout the test period of 6 months, 20 of them were killed for bacteriological examination of the gonads. The testes of 2 cockerels were found to be infected with *E. coli* and in another they harboured *M. gallisepticum* in pure culture. The testes from the other 17 cockerels were sterile. *E. coli* obtained from 20 cockerels were phage typed at the beginning

The phage types were (O)—6, 83, 91, 108, 140 and (H)—1, 6, 8, 10, 25.

Table II (Experiment 2) presents the results of the contamination of the oviducts following repeated insemination with semen only. More frequent inseminations resulted in more contamination. The different parts of the oviducts were contaminated to variable degrees—the uterus most often (15 times), the infundibulum 12 times, magnum 9, isthmus and ovaries 7 and the follicles only 4 times. Cultures of the oviducts of the hens in the control group were sterile.

Table III (Experiment 3) shows the rate of contamination of the oviducts following insemination with semen to which either

E. coli or group D Streptococci were added. Inseminations with larger doses of E. coli (50×10^6) resulted in contamination of 6 out of 10 hens. One out of 10 hens was found to have a contaminated oviduct in each of the groups receiving the lower levels of E. coli ($1 \cdot 0 \times 10^6$ and 10×10^6).

proteus sp., C. albicans and Strep. alpha haemolyticus resulted in 1/6, 2/6, 0/6 and 1/6 contaminations, respectively. The control group remained sterile.

The determinations of pH in the various sections of the oviduct in all the experiments carried out did not show significant changes

TABLE II

CONTAMINATION OF THE OVIDUCT FOLLOWING REPEATED INSEMINATION WITH SEMEN

Group	No. of hens	No. of inseminations	Total vol. of semen inseminated	Number of contaminations						No. of infected hens per group
				Uterus	Isthmus	Magnum	Infundib.	Follicles	Ovary	
1—	6	4	0·2	1C			1C			2/6
2—	6	6	0·3		1C		1C			2/6
3—	30	10	0·5	3C 1C+SD	3C	2C 1C+SD	3C 1SD	2C	2C 2SD	9/10
4—	10	20	1	1S	1S	1S	2S			5/10
5—	10	30	1·5	1C 4SD	1SD	2SD	1C 1SD			5/10
6—	10	40	2	2C 1SD 1PS	2C	1C 1SD	2C	2C	2C 1SD	6/10
Control 7—	6	40	2*	—	—	—	—	—	—	—

* Control group received Ringer's saline solution only.
C—*Escherichia coli.*   SD—Group D streptococci.   S—*Streptococcus alpha haemolyticus.*
PS—*Pseudomonas aeruginosa.*   C+SD—mixed contamination with *Esch. coli* and Group D streptococci.

Group D streptococci contaminated 3 out of 10 oviducts with the larger doses (50×10^6) while the other doses ($1 \cdot 0 \times 10^6$ and 10×10^6) contaminated 1 out of 10 oviducts respectively. The control Group 7 receiving semen only had a higher oviduct contamination rate than the hens of Group 6 receiving an additional 50 million group D streptococci.

Table IV (Experiment 4) represents the capacity of various organisms to contaminate the oviduct of the hen when introduced into the uterus without semen. While group D streptococci contaminated the oviducts of 3 out of 6 hens, Esch. coli, klebsiella sp.,

which could be correlated with the bacterial contamination of the organ.

DISCUSSION

Bacterial contamination of cockerel semen obtained by the milking procedure was first reported by Smith (1949). Although the primary source of the organisms is intestinal, it has been shown in the present work that E. coli and M. gallisepticum can be found in the testes and semen of some cockerels for a period of 6 months. These preliminary findings suggest that testes infected with MG might be an additional means by which infection could be transmitted to the hatching eggs and embryos.

The isolation of *MG* from only 3 of the 464 semen samples could be related to the

TABLE III

CONTAMINATION OF THE OVIDUCT FOLLOWING REPEATED INSEMINATION 15 TIMES AT 4-DAY INTERVALS WITH *E. coli* AND GROUP D STREPTOCOCCI IN ADDITION TO SEMEN

Group	No. of hens	Micro-organisms added to semen	Uterus	Isthmus	Magnum	Infundib.	Follicles	Ovary	No. of infected hens per group
1—	10	*Escherichia coli* 1 × 10⁶	1C						1/10
2—	10	*Escherichia coli* 10 × 10⁶	1C						1/10
3—	10	*Escherichia coli* 50 × 10⁶	6C	3C	1C	3C	1C	2C	6/10
4—	10	group D Streptococci 1× 10⁶	1SD						1/10
5—	10	group D Streptococci 10× 10⁶	1SD						1/10
6—	10	group D Streptococci 50× 10⁶	2SD		1SD				3/10
7—	10	Semen only	1C 2SD	2SD		1C		1C 2SD	4/10
8—	10	Ringer's saline solution only	STERILE						

C—*Escherichia coli*. SD—group D streptococci.

TABLE IV

CONTAMINATION OF THE OVIDUCT FOLLOWING 10 REPEATED INTRAUTERINE INJECTIONS OF VARIOUS MICRO-ORGANISMS

Group	No. of hens	Intrauterine injections	Uterus	Isthmus	Magnum	Infundib.	Follicles	Ovary	No. of infected hens per group
1—	6	*Escherichia coli* 0·5 × 10⁶			1C	1C			1/6
2—	6	Klebsiella sp. 0·5 × 10⁶	1K		1K	1K			2/6
3—	6	Proteus sp. 0·5 × 10⁶	STERILE						0/6
4—	6	*Candida albicans* 0·5 × 10⁶	STERILE						0/6
5—	6	Group D streptococci 0·5 × 10⁶	2SD	1SD	1SD	1SD		3SD	3/6
6—	6	*Streptococcus alpha haemolyticus* 0·5 × 10⁶						1S	1/6
7—	6	Ringer's saline	STERILE						0/6

C—*Escherichia coli*. K—Klebsiella sp. SD—Group D streptococci. S—*Streptococcus alpha haemolyticus*.

fact that the cockerels used in the tests were already mature when selected for their vigour and good health. It is probable that other cockerels were infected with *MG* when young, but intensive antibiotic treatments practised on the farms may have overcome the infection. It is not thought, therefore, that the cockerel plays a major role in the dissemination of this disease.

Bacterial counts of the semen showed a variation of 10^1-10^6 per ml. in 250 samples examined. Following 2 to 3 months of A.I. a decline in fertility has been reported from the field on some farms, but on others not until after 5 to 6 months. It is possible that the better hygienic conditions on some of the farms are responsible for the delay in the decline of fertility; however, in these experiments bacteriological examination of the feed and litter were not carried out in order to investigate this point.

There would appear to be a linear correlation between the number of repeated inseminations of hens and the number of contaminated oviducts (Table II). A further correlation appears to exist between the number of *E. coli* cells in the semen and the number of contaminated oviducts (Table III). Also, the addition of a large number of group D streptococci to the semen increased oviduct contamination (Table III). On the other hand, when semen only was inseminated, 3/10 hens were contaminated with group D streptococci and 2 of them were contaminated with *E. coli* as well; one additional hen showed contamination with *E. coli* only. From this last experiment it might be suggested that when large numbers of *E. coli* or group D streptococci were present in the semen they overwhelmed and suppressed the other organisms so that a pure culture resulted in the oviducts.

The rate of oviduct contamination following repeated administration into the uterus of different organisms without semen (Table IV) showed that group D streptococci were the most active, reaching and infecting the ovary in 3 out of 6 of the hens treated. Neither proteus sp. nor *C. albicans* established infection in this experiment.

ACKNOWLEDGMENTS

The authors wish to acknowledge the support of this investigation by U.S.D.A. Grant No. FG-Is-196.

REFERENCES

Bergey's Manual of Determinative Bacteriology. (1957). Bailliére, Tindall & Cox, London.
BURROWS, W. H., & QUINN, J. P. (1930) U S.D.A. circ. No. 525.
COOPER, D. M. (1955). *Vet. Rec.*, 67, 461.
DEIBEL, R. H. (1964). *Bacteriol. Rev.*, 28, 330.
EDWARDS, P. R., & EWING, W. H. (1964). Identification of Enterobacteriaceae. Burgess Publ. Co., Minnesota.
LUTZENBERG, F. Z., & DOEHL, R. (1956). *Arch. Geflugelz. Kleintierk.*, 6, 241.
PEREK, M. (1966). Physiology of the Domestic Fowl. edit. C. Horton-Smith and E. C. Amoroso, Oliver & Boyd, Edinburgh. p.53-60.
SIMPSON-NOWLAN, S., & DEIBEL, R. H. (1967). *J. Bact.*, 94, 291.
SMITH, A. U. (1949). *J. Agric. Sci.*, 39, 194.
WILSON, G. S., & MILES, A. A. (1964). Topley & Wilson's Principles of Bacteriology and Immunity, Vol. I & II. E. Arnold (Publ.), London.
YODER, Jr., H. W. (1965). Diseases of Poultry—Biester & Schwarte, 5th edition—Iowa State University Press. 405-421.

KEY-WORD TITLE INDEX

AUTHOR INDEX